PREGNANCY
PURE&SIMPLE

Other Avon Books by
Tracie Hotchner

CHILDBIRTH & MARRIAGE
PREGNANCY & CHILDBIRTH
THE PREGNANCY DIARY

TRACIE HOTCHNER

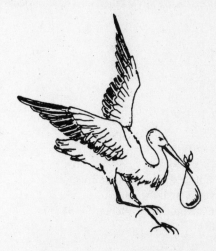

PREGNANCY PURE&SIMPLE

Illustrated by Christine Leahy

AVON BOOKS · NEW YORK

PREGNANCY PURE & SIMPLE is an original publication of Avon Books. This work has never before appeared in book form.

All women, pregnant or otherwise, are strongly advised to consult with their medical caregivers before taking any medications or starting any diet or exercise programs.

AVON BOOKS
A division of
The Hearst Corporation
1350 Avenue of the Americas
New York, New York 10019

Copyright © 1995 by Cortona Corporation
Illustrated by Christine Leahy
Inside cover author photograph by Charles Bush
Published by arrangement with the author
Library of Congress Catalog Card Number: 94-34817
ISBN: 0-380-77434-8

Library of Congress Cataloging in Publication Data:
Hotchner, Tracie
    Pregnancy pure and simple / Tracie Hotchner.
        p.   cm.
    Includes index.
    1. Pregnancy—Popular works.   I. Title.
RG525.H584   1995   94-34817
618.'4—dc20   CIP

First Avon Books Trade Printing: March 1995

AVON TRADEMARK REG. U.S. PAT. OFF. AND IN OTHER COUNTRIES, MARCA REGISTRADA, HECHO EN U.S.A.

Printed in the U.S.A.

ARC   10   9   8   7   6   5   4   3   2   1

This book is dedicated to
my second mother, Peggy,
with love, pure and simple.

Contents

PART III
CHILDBIRTH: PURE AND SIMPLE

PART IV
YOU AND YOUR BABY:
SIMPLY WONDERFUL

A Quick Word
of Introduction

So you're pregnant! Congratulations! You have a great adventure ahead of you. I don't want to bend your ear with a long-winded how-do-you-do because the whole point of this book is to keep things *short and sweet.* You may be familiar with my other pregnancy books, especially *Pregnancy & Childbirth*; that book is often called "the pregnancy bible" by people who've used it. But at 700 pages thick, I realized, it can also be a little intimidating! What if you don't have the time or desire to plow through encyclopedic books that cram your head with more facts than you ever wanted about pregnancy and birth? Or perhaps you *are* interested in a heavy-duty book like *Pregnancy & Childbirth* . . . but you'd also like to have this book to get fast answers (kind of like Cliff Notes for those big books in school!). Turn to any section in *Pregnancy Pure & Simple* and you'll find charts with answers to your concerns. No more scanning through pages of weighty paragraphs, searching for the information you want (some people are already calling this book "Pregnancy Lite").

Pregnancy Pure & Simple is different from other books on the subject because its motto is *Less is more.* I've designed this book for the mother-to-be in the 90s, who needs all the help she can get (and so does her partner in parenting). With two-career couples and the pressures and faster pace of life, starting a family or adding to it can be more complicated today . . . but that doesn't mean that growing a healthy baby and giving birth have to be one more pressure in your life. If you're like many prospective parents today, you don't have much extra time: you want information about your baby that gets right to the point, answering your questions simply yet thoroughly.

This book is "user friendly," with easy-to-find and easy-to-understand bites of information for every stage of your pregnancy. I want to save you the hassle of searching through pages of heavy paragraphs of text when all you want are the plain and simple facts. You'll find everything here you need to have a happy, healthy pregnancy and the birth you want for your baby.

So good luck and have fun on the ultimate adventure you are about to take!

PREGNANCY
PURE&SIMPLE

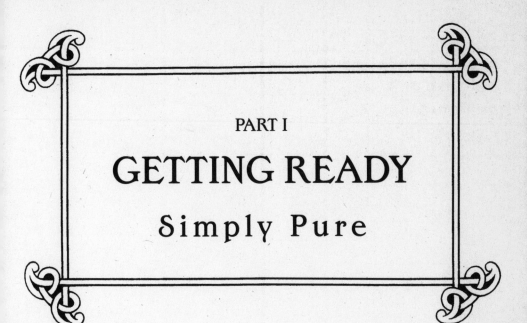

PART I

GETTING READY

Simply Pure

1.
Planning Ahead for a Healthy Pregnancy

Your Health and Things to Avoid

There are many ways for you to prepare yourself and your household for pregnancy before you conceive. Planning ahead can ease the pressure of pregnancy and can mean a healthier baby.

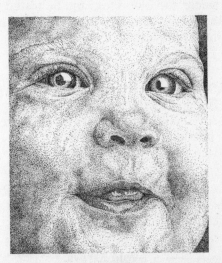

PREPARING YOUR BODY FOR PREGNANCY

GENERAL HEALTH

Have a complete physical examination.
→ Even if you feel fine, it's wise to have a thorough checkup to catch any health problems that might not be treatable during pregnancy.
→ Your partner should make sure he doesn't have any conditions that could interfere with the production or healthiness of his sperm.
→ You should both be tested for sexually transmitted diseases—even if you feel certain you can't possibly be at risk.

Visit the ob/gyn.
→ Before trying to become pregnant have a full examination at your obstetrician.
→ Have a pap smear and blood test, and be tested for vaginal infections. You also need a blood test to check your immunity to rubella (German measles).

Visit the dentist.
→ Pregnancy affects your teeth and gums, so it's a good idea to have a checkup and teeth cleaning.
→ If you need any significant dental work it's better to have it done before becoming pregnant.

See a genetic counselor.
→ If you have any reason to suspect a genetic problem in either of your families, arrange for a genetic screening to ease your minds before conceiving.

Avoid X-rays.
→ Avoid X-rays (other than dental) before conceiving.

Get into shape.

→ If you are overweight, go on a *sensible* diet (preferably monitored by your doctor) so that you're close to your best personal weight when you get pregnant.

→ Avoid crash dieting, which will leave your body deficient of nutrients and vitamins.

→ Develop an exercise routine that fits into your life. Try to get it going before getting pregnant so your body gets used to it.

Put healthy things into your body.

→ Consider drinking only purified water: ordinary tap water has been linked to miscarriage.

→ Get into the habit of eating a well-balanced diet, giving your baby a great start in life.

→ A strict vegetarian diet can affect fertility. Barley, oats, soybeans, carrots, fennel, and green beans are some of the foods that contain natural chemicals that can inhibit fertility.

→ Start taking pregnancy vitamin supplements that contain 0.4 mg. of folic acid *before* you get pregnant.

What to avoid

→ *Avoid alcoholic drinks.*
    ⋘ Don't drink while trying to conceive or during pregnancy.
    ⋘ Alcohol is believed to cause birth defects, mental retardation, and hyperactivity.
    ⋘ See "Alcohol and 'Street Drugs'" on page 10.

→ *Avoid all medications.*
    ⋘ Check with your doctor about any medications you're taking that may interfere with a healthy pregnancy.
    ⋘ Unless you absolutely need them, avoid *any* prescription or over-the-counter medicines.
    ⋘ See "Medications and Stimulants to Avoid" on page 11.

→ *Avoid caffeine.*
    ⋘ High caffeine consumption before and during pregnancy is thought to be linked to miscarriage.
    ⋘ Caffeine can interfere with conception and is linked to birth defects.
    ⋘ See "Caffeine During Pregnancy," page 8, for more information.

→ *Absolutely no "street drugs."*
    ⋘ Any substances that are considered "recreational drugs" are poisonous to your developing baby.
    ⋘ See page 10 for more information.

→ *Stop smoking.*
  - If you can't quit at least cut back as much as possible.
  - See page 7 for more information on ways to quit smoking.

LEAD IN YOUR WATER

* Even at fairly low levels, lead can cause serious developmental problems in the fetus, and health problems for children.
* Before you conceive and during pregnancy, protect yourself from contaminated water.
* If you're going to feed your baby powdered formula, be careful about the water you use to mix it. You might want to use bottled water for greater safety (liquid formula would not pose this problem).

What is a "safe" lead level?
- The Environmental Protection Agency (EPA) says that lead at less than 15 parts per billion can be considered safe.
  - Consumer and environmental groups believe that 10 or even 5 parts per billion is a "better number."
  - Some pediatricians agree with this assessment.
- First get your water tested.
  - Call the EPA toll free at 1-800-426-4791 for the name of state certified laboratories and brochures with more information.
  - A test for lead should cost around $20, although some labs charge as much as $70.
- The testing done when you purchase a house is not sufficient: these tests ordinarily look for bacteria, not lead or other toxic materials.

Well water can be dangerous.
- The problem in houses with wells can come from the pump.
  - Some submersible well pumps are made of lead alloys.
  - These can leak the toxic metal into your household water.
- Millions of Americans use well water: anyone in their fertile years or with small children is advised to have their water tested.

- Homes serviced by public water may also have high lead levels.
- Find out whether lead is coming from your well rather than from the indoor plumbing.
  - ᵃ Take a water sample directly from the containment tank at midmorning.
  - ᵃ Do this by letting the tap run for 30 seconds before taking the sample.
- The U.S. Government has advised that people with new submersible pumps that have lead-alloy parts should drink bottled water.
  - ᵃ Do this as a precaution at least until your water is tested.
  - ᵃ Lab tests have shown that these pumps, especially when they are new, are likely to leak high quantities of lead.

Where's the lead coming from?
- There are a variety of ways that lead can get into your household water.
  - ᵃ It isn't always easy to discover the source of this lead.
  - ᵃ You may need the advice of a home inspector.
- If you have public water, it may pass through lead-pipe service lines from the town's water mains.
- In older houses the problem can be from the pipes, which may have lead or solder with a high lead content.
- Lead can accumulate overnight while the water sits in indoor plumbing.
- Faucets frequently contain lead, even in newer houses. The manufacturer should be able to provide you with data on the amount of lead leaked by their product.

What to do to protect yourself from lead
→ If testing shows that lead occurs consistently only in the "first draw" water (from a tap where the water has rested overnight) then usually the advice is to run the faucet for a full minute before using the water.
→ To make sure no one drinks first-draw water or uses it for cooking, keep a pitcher of "safe" water in the refrigerator.
→ You might want to consider replacing a well pump that contains lead alloys.
→ If the amount of lead in your water is high and can't be traced to other parts of the plumbing in your house, it's easy to find plastic or stainless steel pumps.

Getting the lead out

→ There is a variety of filters available that can remove most of the lead from drinking water: the cost ranges from $100 to $1,000.

→ Surveys of water filters determined that the most effective ones are the reverse-osmosis type, which are expensive.

→ However these can be a good investment when:
  • the lead levels are especially high (above 15 parts per billion),
               OR
  • you are pregnant,
               OR
  • there are small children in the household.

→ Simple filters and distillers, including counter-top models or those that attach to faucets, may be sufficient if the lead level is low.

SMOKING
DURING
PREGNANCY

* For your own health, as well as the health of your baby, now is the time to stop smoking.
* Studies show that smoking while you are pregnant cuts down the oxygen supply to your baby and can cause low birth weight and a generally less healthy baby.
* Give your child a good start in life: if you can't quit entirely then try these suggestions to smoke less.

WAYS TO QUIT SMOKING
OR CUT DOWN

❖ Change to the lowest-tar, lowest-nicotine brand.

❖ Buy only one pack at a time.

❖ Smoke cigarettes only halfway down: tar and nicotine are concentrated nearer the filter.

❖ Keep your cigarettes out of easy reach: make it a conscious effort to get them.

❖ Avoid friends who smoke; it's a contagious habit.

❖ Gradually cut down on the number of cigarettes you smoke.

❖ Smoking for oral gratification could be avoided by munching on low-fat snacks.

❖ When you get the urge for a smoke but want to resist it, try taking a deep breath, holding it, and then letting it out.

❖ If you really want to stop there are plenty of programs available. Ask your doctor's advice.

CAFFEINE DURING PREGNANCY

* Some studies suggest that caffeine may cause reproductive problems like miscarriage, fetal death, and stillbirth.
* High caffeine consumption is considered more than three cups of coffee a day (or the equivalent).
* In the month *before* pregnancy there is also a risk of miscarriage if you consume a lot of caffeine.
* Try to eliminate or reduce your caffeine consumption, especially when trying to conceive and in the first three months of pregnancy.
* The most cautious approach is to assume there is no really safe level of caffeine during pregnancy.

WAYS TO CUT DOWN ON CAFFEINE

✦ Switch to decaffeinated tea and coffee.
✦ Don't let tea steep too long because that increases the caffeine content.
✦ Notice which sodas have high caffeine and switch brands accordingly.
✦ Avoid medications with caffeine (see page 9).

NOTE: When you stop caffeine you may experience a headache that lasts one to seven days—this is a normal reaction to withdrawal from this potent ingredient.

HOW MUCH CAFFEINE IS IN IT?

MILLIGRAMS OF CAFFEINE

Coffee (5 oz.)

automatic drip	110–150
percolated	65–125
instant	40–110
decaffeinated	2–5

Tea (5 oz.)

5-minute brew	50–90
3-minute brew	20–45
canned iced tea (12 oz.)	25–35
decaffeinated	0

Chocolate

cocoa beverage	10
milk chocolate (1 oz.)	6
baking chocolate (1 oz.)	35

Soft drinks (12 oz.), diet or regular

Mountain Dew, Mr. Pibb, Mellow Yellow	53
Sunkist Orange (diet is 0)	42
Coca-Cola, Tab, Shasta Cola	45
Pepsi, Dr Pepper, RC Cola	35
Diet-Rite	35
7-Up, Sprite, Root Beer, Fresca, ginger ale	0

Nonprescription medications (standard dose)

Anacin, Midol	64
Excedrin	130
plain aspirin (any brand)	0
Dexatrim, Dietac	200
No Doz, Vivarin, Caffedrine	200
Dristan, Coryban-D	30

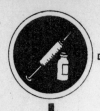
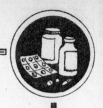

ALCOHOL AND "STREET DRUGS"

Hard liquor, wine, and beer
- There is no "safe" amount of alcohol—can cause physical defects, learning defects and emotional problems.
- More than two ounces of hard liquor a day can permanently harm your developing baby.
- Drinking excessively *even one time* can cause "fetal alcohol syndrome," which results in permanent physical and behavioral abnormalities in your child.
- It is best to avoid alcohol altogether during pregnancy.

Amphetamines ("uppers," "speed")
- These drugs are dangerous stimulants to the baby's nervous system.

Cocaine and crack
- Can kill your baby.
- Can cause a baby to be born addicted, suffering a painful withdrawal at birth.
- Cocaine causes long-term behavioral, neurological, and developmental problems.

Heroin, morphine
- Can cause fetal addiction, which means an agonizing withdrawal at birth.
- A baby may need a blood transfusion at birth.

LSD and other psychedelics
- Increase the risk of miscarriage.
- May also cause chromosomal damage to your unborn child.

Marijuana
- Smoking even moderate quantities of grass can cause fertility problems, complicated pregnancies, and low-birth-weight babies.
- Can also cause stillbirth and early infant death.

Tranquilizers (Quaaludes and other "downers")
- May cause deformities in the first trimester.

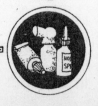

Medications

**Accutane
(isotretinoin)**
- An acne drug that causes severe and often lethal birth defects.
- Do not take this medication during your childbearing years; even one pill can be devastating.

Ace inhibitors
- Commonly given for high blood pressure.
- Causes deformities or fetal death in the second and third trimester.
- If you've been on an Ace inhibitor, talk to your doctor about alternatives.
- Don't just stop taking medications: there could be serious danger to you and your baby.

Aerosol ribavirin
- Used to treat severe lung infections in young children.
- For health-care workers who handle it, breathing the mist can lead to birth defects.

**Anabolic drugs
(steroids)**
- Used for bodybuilding to add weight and muscle.
- They should be avoided during pregnancy.

Anesthetic gases
- Suspected to be the cause of high rates of sterility, miscarriage, and birth defects among hospital personnel exposed to the gases.

Antibiotics
- Some antibiotics can cross the placenta and cause birth defects or even death.
- Check with your doctor about any antibiotic to make sure it cannot harm your developing baby.

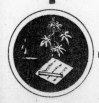

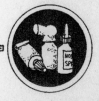

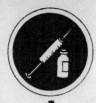

Anticonvulsants (Dilantin, etc.)	■ Can cause abnormalities like cleft lip and cleft palate. ■ If stopping the anticonvulsant would be dangerous to your health, folic acid may counteract the possibility of birth defects.
Antihistamines	■ Causes malformations in the baby. ■ Check with your doctor about antihistamines that have been designed for safe use during pregnancy.
Antimetabolites (antitumor drugs)	■ Medications like aminopterin can cause malformations of the fetus.
Antinausea drugs	■ Have caused malformations in the offspring of test animals. ■ Avoid if possible or talk to your doctor.
Aspirin	■ Can cause miscarriage when taken in large amounts. ■ Frequent use toward the end of pregnancy may cause the newborn to hemorrhage. ■ Aspirin affects your blood-clotting mechanisms. This can be fatal during labor and delivery.
Birth control pills	■ Can cause fetal malformations.
Blood-pressure-lowering drugs	■ See "Ace inhibitors" and "Reserpine."
Cancer chemotherapy	■ A high risk of miscarriages for pregnant nurses who handle them during the first trimester. ■ Health-care professionals who are pregnant or trying to conceive should avoid exposure to these medications.
Cortisone	■ Can cause abnormalities or stillbirth.

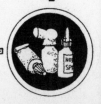

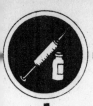

Cough syrup	■ Especially dangerous early in the development of the baby.
	■ Even over-the-counter brands are not recommended.
Diet pills (dextroamphetamines)	■ Can cause heart defects and blood vessel malformations.
Diuretics (water pills)	■ Causes blood disorders or jaundice in the newborn.
Haldol (haloperidol)	■ A tranquilizer used in treating schizophrenia.
	■ Can permanently alter the baby's brain chemistry.
	■ However, schizophrenia runs in families and is thought to have a genetic component. If a baby at risk for schizophrenia receives haloperidol via its mother before birth it might decrease the chance of developing the illness later in life.
	■ Discuss risk versus advantage with your doctor.
Iodides (expectorants)	■ Can cause a goiter in an unborn child.
Nose drops and sprays	■ Can be strong enough to contract blood vessels in the placenta, reducing oxygen and nutrition carried to the fetus.
Phenacetin	■ Causes possible damage to the developing kidneys.
Progestins (progesteronelike hormones)	■ Linked to birth defects, particularly genital defects in females.
Reserpine	■ Drugs to lower blood pressure can cause blood disorders and jaundice in newborns.

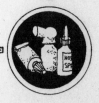

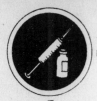
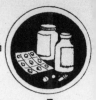

Sulfa drugs
- Taken in late pregnancy, they can disturb a baby's liver function and produce a form of jaundice associated with brain damage.

Tegison (etretinate)
- Used to treat severe cases of psoriasis.
- Even after it is discontinued, this drug stays in a person's body for two years.
- Tegison can continue to cause severe birth defects long after you stop taking it.

Thyroid medications
- Can cause goiter in the infant.

Tranquilizers
- May cause deformities in the first trimester.
- Check with your ob/gyn for tranquilizers designed for safe use during pregnancy.

Vitamins
- Can be dangerous if used in excess quantities.
- See following section and chart "Vitamins Can Be Dangerous," page 22.

NOTE: If you have any questions about any other medications and your doctor does not have the answers, contact the March of Dimes. The national office is at 1275 Mamaroneck Avenue, White Plains, New York 10605. There may also be a local office in your area.

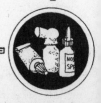

VITAMINS REALLY MATTER

* The food you eat is the best possible source of vitamins—but you can't be sure of the vitamin content of the ingredients (especially if you eat out frequently).
* It's hard to eat a carefully balanced diet every single day, especially with a busy schedule and/or nausea.
* Maybe you don't think you need to take vitamins if you're eating the right healthy foods? But no matter how conscientious you are, no diet can supply the amounts of *iron* (explained on pages 20–21) and *folic acid* that are necessary for a healthy baby.
* Folic acid (also called "folacin") is one of the B vitamins essential to a successful pregnancy: your body needs twice as much of it now. Deficiencies during pregnancy are common and can result in miscarriage or damage to the unborn child.

> **WARNING: If you were taking the birth control pill until shortly before you conceived, a folic acid deficiency is likely. The supplement is even more important for you.**

* Vitamin supplements are included in prenatal care because you need at least these basic vitamin necessities for pregnancy:
  * iron (60 mg.)
  * folic acid (0.8 mg.)
  * calcium (1,200 mg.)
  * vitamin A (6,000 I.U.)
  * vitamin D (400 I.U.)
* You have to take a vitamin supplement *every day* because the body cannot store many of these elements.
* Don't make the mistake of thinking that if a vitamin is good, more of it will be better: there is a danger in taking large amounts of vitamins. For example, the body does not excrete vitamins A and D. Also, any vitamin taken in excessive amounts can cause birth defects (see the "warnings" box on page 22 after the following Vitamin Directory).

VITAMIN DIRECTORY

Vitamin A

Foods
- fortified whole milk
- fortified margarine
- butter
- egg yolk
- fish liver oils
- liver and kidney
- deep green and yellow vegetables (cooked vegetables provide A more readily than raw ones)

Daily requirement
- 6,000 I.U. during pregnancy
- 8,000 I.U. when breast-feeding

What it does
- builds resistance to infection
- functions in vision
- helps formation of tooth enamel, hair, and fingernails
- necessary for proper growth and function of the thyroid gland

Vitamin B

(includes all vitamins B_1 through B_{12}, including niacin)

Foods
- brewer's yeast:
  - purchase at a health food store
  - start out with a teaspoon in juice and build up to one tablespoon
  - do not use live yeast
- bread
- whole grains
- wheat germ
- liver

What it does
- prevents nervousness
- helps skin problems
- provides energy
- prevents constipation

16

B₁ (thiamin)

Foods
- pork and pork products
- liver, heart, and kidney
- peas and beans
- wheat germ

Daily requirement
- 1.2 mg. in pregnancy
- 1.5 mg. while breast-feeding

What it does
- essential for appetite and digestion
- needed for fertility, growth, and breast-feeding
- needed during illness and infection

B₂ (riboflavin)

Foods
- milk—each quart contains 2 mg.

Daily requirement
- 5 to 10 mg.

What it does
- necessary for normal growth and development of the baby from conception

Niacin

Foods
- liver
- beef
- poultry
- tuna
- milk
- peanuts and almonds
- brown rice
- wheat
- peas

Daily requirement
- 20 to 50 mg.

What it does
- prevents infections and bleeding of gums

B₆ (pyridoxine)

Foods
- yeast
- liver
- wheat germ

- whole-grain bread
- cereal
- green beans and leafy green vegetables
- bananas
- meat and fish
- nuts
- potatoes

Daily requirement
- 2 to 20 mg.

What it does
- essential for the metabolism of fats
- produces antibodies that fight disease

B_{12} (cobalamin)

Foods
- yeast
- liver
- wheat germ
- whole grains
- kidneys
- meat and fish
- eggs
- milk
- oysters

Daily requirement
- 8 to 15 mg.

What it does
- essential for development of red blood cells

Vitamin C

Foods
- citrus fruits
- cantaloupe
- strawberries
- green and red bell peppers
- broccoli
- cauliflower
- tomatoes
- potatoes
  (Overcooking or cooking vegetables in too much water destroys the vitamin C. Ascorbic acid [synthetic] is identical to natural vitamin C.)

Daily requirement
- 80 mg. minimum
- Do not exceed 1 gram.
- Stress, alcohol, smoking, the Pill, and aspirin all interfere with absorption and levels in the body.
- Smokers require larger amounts, about 25 mg. per cigarette.
- Ascorbic acid (synthetic) is identical to natural vitamin C.

What it does
- helps the body resist infection

Calcium

Foods
- milk
- stone-ground grains
- vitamin C helps in absorption

Daily requirement
- 1,200 mg.
- Pregnant women give more calcium to the baby than they're taking in.
- For better absorption take calcium gluconate or calcium lactate pills on an empty stomach with sour milk, yogurt, or an acid fruit or juice.

What it does
- builds baby's bones and teeth

Vitamin D

Foods
- vitamin D–fortified milk
- fish liver oils
- mackerel, salmon, tuna, sardines, and herring
- Another source is sunshine.

Daily requirement
- 400 I.U.
- Varies with exposure to the sun and your complexion: dark-skinned people need more sun to manufacture vitamin D.

What it does
- helps absorption of calcium from the blood into tissue and bone cells

Vitamin E

Foods
- whole grains
- corn
- peanuts
- eggs

Daily requirement
- 30 mg.

What it does
- governs the amount of oxygen the body uses
- promotes healing

Folic Acid

Foods
- liver
- leafy green vegetables
- broccoli and asparagus
- peanuts

Daily requirement
- 800 micrograms (0.8 mg.) (The body does not store folic acid so 0.8 mg. *must* be taken every day.)

What it does
- essential for blood formation and formation of new cells

Iodine

Foods
- iodized salt

Daily requirement
- season food to taste with iodized salt

What it does
- helps thyroid gland function properly, regulating your metabolism

Iron

Food
- liver (or liver pills, if you hate liver)
- fish and meat
- egg yolks
- raisins
- dark molasses

Daily requirement	■ 30 to 60 mg.
	■ Many young women are iron-deficient before pregnancy.
	■ More iron is needed in the second half of pregnancy.
What it does	■ Iron is the main component of blood hemoglobin that carries oxygen to the baby and your cells.
	■ The baby draws on your supply to store iron in its liver to carry it through its milk diet during the first four to six months of independent life.

Vitamin K

Foods	■ Vitamin K doesn't come directly from food— it's synthesized by stomach bacteria.
Daily requirement	■ For baby: a vitamin K injection is usually given to babies at birth to guard against hemorrhage.
What it does	■ necessary for normal blood clotting

Zinc

Foods	■ seafood
	■ liver
	■ beets
	■ barley
	■ carrots
	■ cabbage
Daily requirement	■ minimum 15 mg.
What it does	■ promotes healthy function of organs
	■ promotes wound healing

VITAMINS CAN BE DANGEROUS

Vitamins in large doses can be dangerous to your developing baby.

VITAMIN	DANGER	SAFE DAILY AMOUNT
A	✤ In excess, vitamin A may cause birth defects.	under 6,000 I.U.
B$_6$ (pyridoxine)	✤ Can cause nerve problems in mother.	under 200 mg.
C	✤ May impair fetal bone development. Can cause scurvy in newborn.	under 1 gram
	✤ Vitamin C is an active metabolic agent: the full effect of large doses on the fetus is not known.	
D	✤ Can cause mental retardation, heart defects, or bone defects in the baby.	under 400 I.U.
E	✤ Raises blood pressure in people not accustomed to it.	under 800 I.U.
	✤ Restricted intake for women with high blood pressure or a rheumatic heart condition.	under 150 I.U.
K	✤ Can cause jaundice, which may damage the baby's nervous system.	Available by prescription only.

WHEN TO STOP USING BIRTH CONTROL

* Many birth control methods pose some risk to the baby even after you've stopped using them.
* You should be aware of these risks before you attempt to get pregnant.
* In the meantime the safest method of birth control is the condom.

DANGERS OF PREVIOUS BIRTH CONTROL METHODS

Birth control pill
+ Can cause birth defects
+ Discontinue use for 3 months or 2 menstrual cycles

IUD
+ Possibility of miscarriage or premature birth if left in place after conception
+ Remove before attempting pregnancy or as soon as you know you are pregnant

Spermicides (cream, jelly, foam, etc.)
+ May be linked to birth defects or miscarriage
+ Stop using about 1 month before trying to conceive

Diaphragm
+ Used with spermicides, has possible risks as above
+ Stop using at least 1 month before

DANGERS TO A FATHER'S SPERM

If a father-to-be is exposed to toxic substances before conceiving a child there may be risks to the fetus.

Vitamin C deficiency
✢ Taking in less than the recommended 60 mg. a day can damage sperm and increase infertility. A deficiency can also cause birth defects.

Exposure to toxins in the workplace
✢ Benzene, X-rays, and some art and textile chemicals are hazardous.
✢ Can cause premature births, low birth weight, or stillborn infants.

Exposure to electromagnetic fields
✢ Applies to men in jobs like electricians, power line repairmen, and welders.
✢ One study shows these workers are twelve times as likely to have a baby who develops a neuroblastoma.

Regular exposure to paints
✢ Increases the risk of a child's developing a brain tumor before age ten.

Smoking
✢ A father who smokes before conception increases the chance of his child's developing leukemia by 40 percent.

Drinking alcohol
✢ Drinking more than two alcoholic drinks daily in the month before conception can result in his child's being 5 ounces lighter than the average.

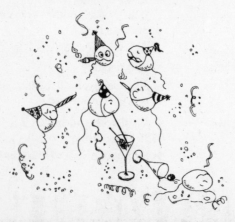

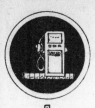

EVERYDAY HAZARDS

Aerosol sprays
- Inhaling the fumes can be harmful to the developing baby.
- Use pump sprays instead.

Air pollution
- Carbon monoxide from car exhaust fumes can cause low birth weight.
- Avoid walking and jogging around traffic.
- Don't drive with your windows open in heavy traffic.
- Keep the air vent on "recirculate."

Anesthetic gases
- Encountered in high amounts by all health personnel in operating rooms.
- These professionals have abnormally high rates of sterility, miscarriage, and birth deformities.
- Exposure to these gases is suspected cause.

Cadmium
- A component of tobacco smoke, wastes from electroplating plants, and released by tires burning or wearing down.
- Retards fetal growth, linked to fetal deformities.

Caffeine
- Occurs even in decaffeinated coffee and tea.
- Stimulates fetal nervous system.
- Refer to pages 8–9 for details.

Carbon monoxide
- Avoid driving in traffic jams or in a car in an enclosed space (garage, tunnel).
- Don't walk in areas with heavy traffic.
- Extended exposure can cause low birth weight or infant mortality.
- Vehicle fumes also contain lead, a poisonous gas.

Cat litter box
- Soiled kitty litter carries toxoplasmosis, which can damage the unborn child.
- Have someone else clean the litter box.

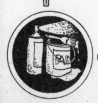
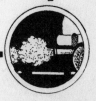

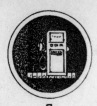
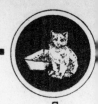

Chemotherapy drugs	■ Certain cancer medications handled by nurses in first trimester cause high risk of miscarriage.
	■ Fetal loss linked to on-the-job exposure to 3 drugs: cyclophosphamide, doxorubicin, and vincristine.
	■ All three drugs stop cancer by disrupting cell growth and killing actively growing cells.
Computer chip factories	■ Studies show a high miscarriage rate for women exposed to chemicals used in making chips.
Fish	■ Can be contaminated by water they live in.
	■ See pages 52–54 for more information.
Food additives	■ Artificial colors, preservatives, growth hormones and antibiotics are dangerous for the developing baby.
	■ See page 51 for more information.
Gasoline	■ Gas vapors can cause cancer and birth defects.
	■ Do not fill your own gas tank. Vapor retrieval hoses can be defective.
Hot tubs	■ High temperatures (over 106°F.) can cause brain damage in the unborn baby.
	■ Keep water below 104 degrees.
	■ Get out after ten minutes to cool off before going back into the hot tub.
Household cleaning products	■ Avoid strong-smelling cleaning products.
	■ Make sure there is adequate ventilation when you're around cleaning agents.
Lawn and garden chemicals	■ Wear gloves and wash your hands after gardening.
	■ Don't breathe the fumes of strong gardening products.

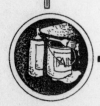

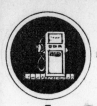

Lead in water	■ Even a small amount causes birth defects and should be strictly avoided. ■ New faucets have very high levels of lead. ■ Old faucets can also leak up to ten years after installation. ■ Reduce the risk of lead by always running tap water for *sixty second*s before using it. ■ A water analysis lab can analyze your water (see pages 4–6).
Lecithin	■ A fat-emulsifying substance sold in health-food stores, often as a diet aid. ■ Damage is possible to the developing fetus: beware during childbearing years.
Mercury	■ May be in medical or industrial compounds as mercurous chloride. ■ Overexposure can cause brain damage, blindness, or cerebral palsy.
Microwave oven	■ There is speculation that microwaves may harm your unborn child. ■ As a precaution, use a meter to find out if your microwave might have a leak.
Ozone	■ An oxygen variant occurring in high concentrations of smog. ■ Can exist in airplanes at high altitudes. ■ Believed to be the cause of high rates of miscarriage and birth defects for flight attendants.
Paints	■ Paint may contain lead or toxic vapors. ■ Avoid areas where old paint is being sanded or old furniture is being refinished. ■ Latex paints are safe.
PCBs	■ Cancer-causing chemicals banned since 1979 but still present in the food chain, especially water supplies. ■ Avoid fresh-water and bottom-feeding fish like flounder and sole. ■ Causes birth defects.

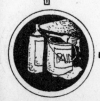

Pesticides
■ Excessive contact with almost any pesti-cides can harm the unborn child.

Photographic chemicals
■ High doses of darkroom chemicals may injure the fetus.
■ Completely avoid these organic and metal-lic chemicals in the first trimester.
■ In the second and third trimester you can work in the darkroom but take precau-tions: wear goggles and impermeable gloves and be sure of adequate ventilation.

Meat, raw or rare
■ This can cause toxoplasmosis (see page 38).

Solvents
■ Substances like turpentine and toluene can be hazardous during pregnancy.
■ Avoid long exposure to constant high con-centrations in industrial arts or crafts.

Tobacco smoke
■ There are toxic substances in tobacco smoke that stunt the baby's growth. (See page 7.)
■ This is true whether you are the smoker or you're inhaling secondary smoke.

Toxic products
■ *Read the label of any product you use during pregnancy.*
■ You must not inhale toxic products (for example: cleaning fluid, contact cement, volatile paint, lacquer thinner, some glues, some household cleaning products like oven cleaner, etc.)

Water
■ Chemicals and lead are present in the public water supply and can cause miscar-riage and birth defects. See page 4 on "Lead in Your Water."
■ Although tap water is "officially safe" you might want to use bottled water for drink-ing and cooking.
■ You could also put a carbon filter on one sink in your house and use only that for cooking and drinking.

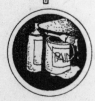

Uranium wastes
- Radioactive material from mining was used in Colorado to build roads and house foundations.
- Cinder-blocks made of this radioactive slag were used to build homes in many other states.
- Rain that drains through uranium mining waste has made drinking water abnormally radioactive in parts of Colorado, New Mexico, and Utah, etc.
- This heightened radiation increases the incidence of miscarriage and birth defects.

Vaginal products
- Avoid feminine hygiene products like douches and gels containing povidone-iodine.
- During pregnancy this can possibly cause thyroid defects in the baby.

X-rays
- Strictly avoid having X-rays unless they are absolutely necessary.
- Tell the technician you are pregnant beforehand.
- Dental X-rays are safe if you wear an lead apron.

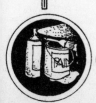

IS YOUR BABY AT RISK?

COOLEY'S ANEMIA

What is it?
- An inherited blood disorder causing anemia in the child.
- Symptoms don't appear until the first or second year of life.
- The child will be pale, listless, and have a poor appetite and frequent infections.
- In severe cases it's necessary for the child to have regular blood transfusions.

Who gets it?
Carriers are of Mediterranean descent, mostly Greek and Italian.

CYSTIC FIBROSIS

What is it?
A genetic disease affecting breathing and digestion.

Who gets it?
- One in twenty Americans is a carrier.
- If either of your parents has/had cystic fibrosis, it is assumed you are a carrier.
- Most carriers are Caucasian.

Can you protect against it?
- Testing of family members may provide a more accurate evaluation of your status, although these tests are not fully dependable.
- Most university hospitals have a genetics department you can contact to do this testing.

NEURAL TUBE DEFECTS (NTDs)

What are they?

- Defects involving the central nervous system and neural tube.
- These birth defects occur by the end of the first month of pregnancy.

Who gets them?

- NTDs occur in one in a thousand births.
- A family history of NTDs increases your risk.

How can you protect against them?

- A pregnant woman's diet may have something to do with NTDs.
- Women taking multivitamin pills before getting pregnant have 50 percent fewer cases of NTDs.
- Use moderation, however, since *large* doses of vitamins are a potential cause of birth defects. (See page 22, "Vitamins Can Be Dangerous.")

RUBELLA (GERMAN MEASLES)

What is it?

- A rash spreading from your face to your body and swollen lymph glands in the neck.
- The disease can cause miscarriage, stillbirth, and birth defects if you are infected by it in the first three months of pregnancy.
- It takes two to three weeks after exposure for the symptoms to appear.

Who gets it?

- If you had German measles (which are not the same as regular measles) as a child, then you are immune.
- If a woman develops rubella while pregnant, there is a one-in-five chance that her fetus will be affected.

Can you protect against it?

- Have a blood test before you get pregnant to find out if you are immune.
- If you are not immune, get inoculated.
- *Do not* get pregnant for three months after the inoculation.
- *Do not get immunized while you are pregnant.* The vaccine can harm the baby.

- Stay away from children one to twelve years old.
- If you come into contact with an infected person while you are pregnant your doctor can give you a shot to prevent you from developing the disease.

RH BLOOD INCOMPATIBILITY

What is it?
- A genetically determined substance in the red blood cells that is missing in some people.
- If a woman is Rh negative and her baby is Rh positive there can be a bad reaction if their blood cells mix.

Who gets it?
- It rarely happens in the first pregnancy.
- If the baby's blood enters the mother's blood at delivery destructive antibodies can develop that will cause problems in later pregnancies.

Can you protect against it?
- All Rh negative women should get a shot of Rh immunoglobulin within seventy-two hours of:
  - the delivery of an Rh positive baby
  - *any* miscarriage or abortion

SICKLE-CELL ANEMIA

What is it?
- A hereditary disease that affects mostly African-Americans.
- It is not apparent at birth.
- Symptoms usually don't occur until after the child is two.
- It can cause death, often from infections, in children who get it early in life.

Who gets it?
- There is an inexpensive test to find out whether you are a carrier or have the disease.
- One out of ten African-Americans carries the trait or has the disease.

- If both parents are carriers the child has a 25 percent chance of having the disease and a 50 percent chance of being a carrier.
- If only one parent is a carrier none of the children will have sickle-cell. However, the children have a 50 percent chance of being carriers.

Can you protect against it?
- There is no way to cure or prevent this disease.
- There is an inexpensive test to find out whether you are a carrier or have the disease.
- A baby with sickle-cell can be diagnosed in the womb.
- The test is a difficult procedure. It should be done only if both parents are carriers and would abort if the baby tested positive for the disease.

TAY-SACHS DISEASE

What is it?
- A crippling, fatal disorder caused by the lack of a specific enzyme.
- A child loses motor abilities; becomes deaf, blind, and retarded; and usually dies before the age of four.

Who gets it?
- Primarily carried by people of Ashkenazi Jewish ancestry: 90 percent of U.S. Jews are of Ashkenazi origin.
- The odds of having a child with the disease are the same with each pregnancy.
- If two carriers marry, each child has a:
  - 25 percent risk of having Tay-Sachs disease
  - 25 percent chance of being totally free of the disease
  - 50 percent chance of being a carrier like the parents

Can you protect against it?
If you think you are at risk, be tested for the disease before you try conceiving—or even before you marry.

WILSON'S DISEASE

What is it?
- A defect in metabolism of copper in the body, causing excess copper in the brain, liver, and eyes.
- Without treatment the illness can cause mental derangement and cirrhosis of the liver.

Who gets it?
- There is no specific group susceptible.
- It is a good idea for everyone to be tested before conceiving.

INFECTIOUS DISEASES
THAT CAN HARM YOUR BABY

HEPATITIS B

What is it?
- An infection caused by a virus. It can be passed to your baby during birth.
- It can cause a severe liver disease.

Who gets it?
- Anyone can get hepatitis.
- You may be a carrier of the virus without any signs of illness.

How can you protect the baby?
If tests are done while you are pregnant your baby can get the necessary treatment at birth to prevent getting the disease.

HERPES SIMPLEX VIRUS

What is it?
- A venereal disease consisting of fluid-filled blisters on any part of the body, usually around the genital area.
- Sometimes there is a fever, headache, and painful urination.
- Herpes is usually noticed three to fourteen days after sexual contact.

How do you get it?
- Sexual contact with someone who has herpes during active recurrence. (The virus is inactive between flare-ups.)
- The virus is passed to the baby through the birth canal when the mother has active vaginal lesions at the time of birth.

How can you protect the baby?

- Medication is available to control herpes. It isn't yet known whether it is safe to use during pregnancy.
- Mental and physical stress can cause recurrence.
- Mothers with a history of herpes should take very good care of themselves. Eat well. Get plenty of sleep. Keep clean and wear loose-fitting underwear.
- A woman with the herpes virus must be examined for recurrent infection as her due date nears.
- If you have herpetic sores in the genital area at the time of delivery the baby must be delivered by cesarean section.

What role does your diet play?

- Diet therapy has been suggested as a way to control herpes.
- Following this diet has not been proven to be a help, but it does indicate that manipulating your diet may help.
- Foods rich in L-lysine can stop the growth of herpes while foods high in arginine promote infection.
- Talk to your doctor about supplementing your diet with L-lysine supplement, available in health food stores.
- Any woman with a history of herpes should avoid arginine-rich foods for the last six weeks of pregnancy.

HERPES AND WHAT YOU EAT

FOODS TO EAT (Lysine-rich)	FOODS TO AVOID (Arginine-rich)
Fish and chicken	Nuts and seeds
Beef and lamb	Brown rice and corn
Milk and dairy products	Oatmeal
Beans	Chocolate, cocoa, carob
Brewer's yeast	Coconut and raisins
Shellfish	Gelatin
Eggs	Buckwheat and whole wheat flour

LISTERIOSIS

What is it?

- The listeria bacteria causes a potentially fatal intestinal infection.
- Although it's rarely mentioned, it can cause early miscarriage, premature labor, or stillbirth.
- If the baby survives listeriosis, there can be damage to the lungs, brain, kidneys, and liver.

Who gets it?

Pregnant women are especially susceptible to the type of bacteria that causes this disease.

How can you protect your baby?

- The listeria bacteria is widespread in the food supply.
- It is important that pregnant women use caution when preparing food.

WAYS TO PREVENT LISTERIOSIS

✤ Avoid raw milk or foods made from raw milk.

✤ Wash hands, knives, cutting boards, and counter surfaces after they come in contact with uncooked foods.

✤ Wash raw vegetables thoroughly.

✤ Keep uncooked meats separate from vegetables and cooked foods.

✤ Keep refrigerators clean and cold (34–40°F.).

✤ Avoid soft cheese like Brie, Camembert, feta, and blue-veined cheese.

✤ Leftovers or ready-to-eat-foods like hot dogs should be fully reheated until steaming hot.

✤ Avoid luncheon meats from delicatessen counters or thoroughly reheat them before eating.

TOXOPLASMOSIS

What is it?
- A disease caused by a parasite that is passed on to humans by eating raw meat or having contact with cat feces.
- Causes neurological problems in the unborn child.
- Baby can appear normal at birth but may develop symptoms later.

Who gets it?
- You may be immune to this disease because one third of women have already been exposed to toxoplasmosis.
- Your chances of being immune increase if you have eaten raw or rare meat or have been caring for cats.
- The greatest danger of infecting the fetus is in the last months of pregnancy.

How can you protect your baby?
- A blood test can tell whether you're immune. However, the test is not entirely reliable, and must be repeated to confirm accuracy.
- The suggestions below can help protect you against the disease.

WAYS TO PREVENT TOXOPLASMOSIS

- ✤ Don't eat raw or rare meat. Cook meat to at least 140 degrees.
- ✤ Wash hands thoroughly after handling raw meat.
- ✤ Have your cat(s) tested to see if they have an active infection. If they test positive, board them at a vet or at a friend's house during your pregnancy.
- ✤ Don't handle cat litter.
- ✤ Do not feed rare or raw food to your cats. Infected meat (mice, birds, etc.) is the carrier.
- ✤ Avoid other people's cats, especially outdoor cats.

2.

Eating to Make a Healthy Baby

The Good and the Bad

You can start being a responsible, loving mother from the first day you find out you are pregnant: eat well for your growing baby. There is nothing more important you can do for him in the next nine months than to take care of your own body and nourish the baby with safe and nutritious foods.

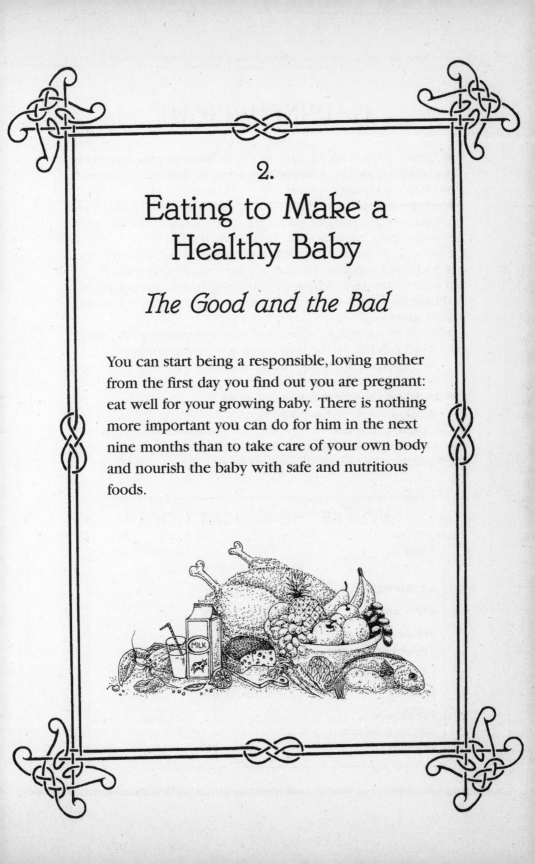

GAINING WEIGHT

* Pregnant women are often concerned about gaining too much weight but you'll stop worrying once you understand where the pounds are going.
* Once you've seen it spelled out in pounds why and how you're gaining weight you can eat lots of good food without any guilt because your baby and your body need the fuel!
* From about the twelfth week of pregnancy you'll probably see a noticeable change on the scales when you weigh yourself.
* If you're eating sensibly, most of the weight you are gaining is the baby—for most women it's about 40 percent of the weight they gain.
* The rest of the weight you gain during pregnancy works out at:
    * 22 percent for the increase in your blood volume
    * 8 percent for your enhanced breasts
    * 10 percent for the uterus
    * 10 percent for the amniotic fluid
    * 10 percent for the placenta
* The chart below shows how the minimum you will gain is around 20 pounds, although your weight gain can be as much as 35 pounds and still be within this range.

WHERE THE WEIGHT GOES

Baby	7 1/2 to 8 1/2 pounds (average newborn weight)
Amniotic fluid	1 to 2 pounds
Placenta	1 to 2 pounds
Mother's blood and body fluids	increase by 4 to 8 pounds
Uterine muscles	2 to 3 pounds
Breasts	enlarge by 2 to 3 pounds
Fat deposits (around internal organs)	2 to 10 pounds

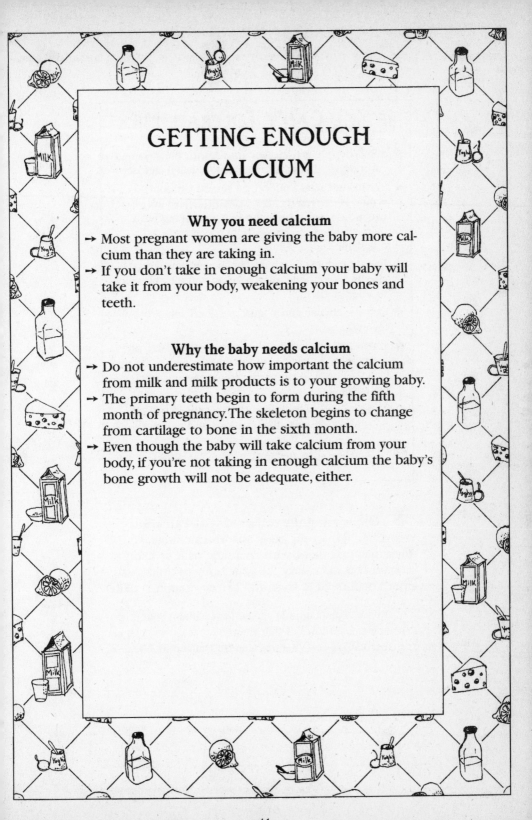

GETTING ENOUGH CALCIUM

Why you need calcium

→ Most pregnant women are giving the baby more calcium than they are taking in.
→ If you don't take in enough calcium your baby will take it from your body, weakening your bones and teeth.

Why the baby needs calcium

→ Do not underestimate how important the calcium from milk and milk products is to your growing baby.
→ The primary teeth begin to form during the fifth month of pregnancy. The skeleton begins to change from cartilage to bone in the sixth month.
→ Even though the baby will take calcium from your body, if you're not taking in enough calcium the baby's bone growth will not be adequate, either.

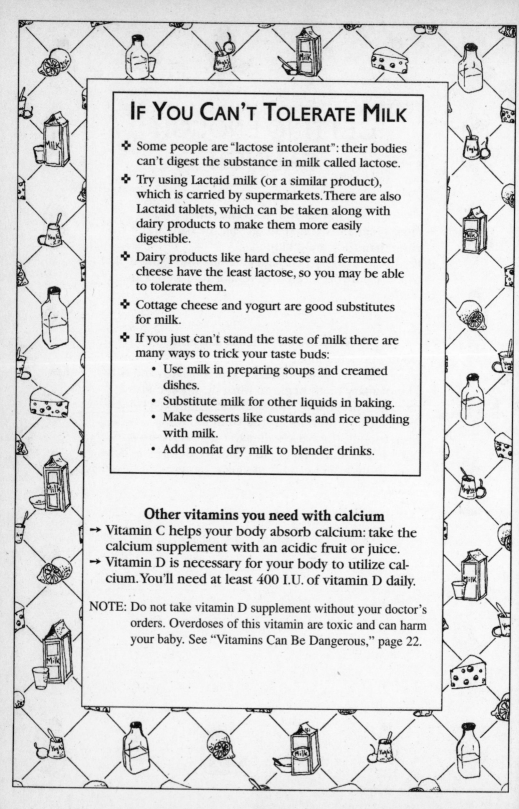

IF YOU CAN'T TOLERATE MILK

✤ Some people are "lactose intolerant": their bodies can't digest the substance in milk called lactose.

✤ Try using Lactaid milk (or a similar product), which is carried by supermarkets. There are also Lactaid tablets, which can be taken along with dairy products to make them more easily digestible.

✤ Dairy products like hard cheese and fermented cheese have the least lactose, so you may be able to tolerate them.

✤ Cottage cheese and yogurt are good substitutes for milk.

✤ If you just can't stand the taste of milk there are many ways to trick your taste buds:
  • Use milk in preparing soups and creamed dishes.
  • Substitute milk for other liquids in baking.
  • Make desserts like custards and rice pudding with milk.
  • Add nonfat dry milk to blender drinks.

Other vitamins you need with calcium

→ Vitamin C helps your body absorb calcium: take the calcium supplement with an acidic fruit or juice.

→ Vitamin D is necessary for your body to utilize calcium. You'll need at least 400 I.U. of vitamin D daily.

NOTE: Do not take vitamin D supplement without your doctor's orders. Overdoses of this vitamin are toxic and can harm your baby. See "Vitamins Can Be Dangerous," page 22.

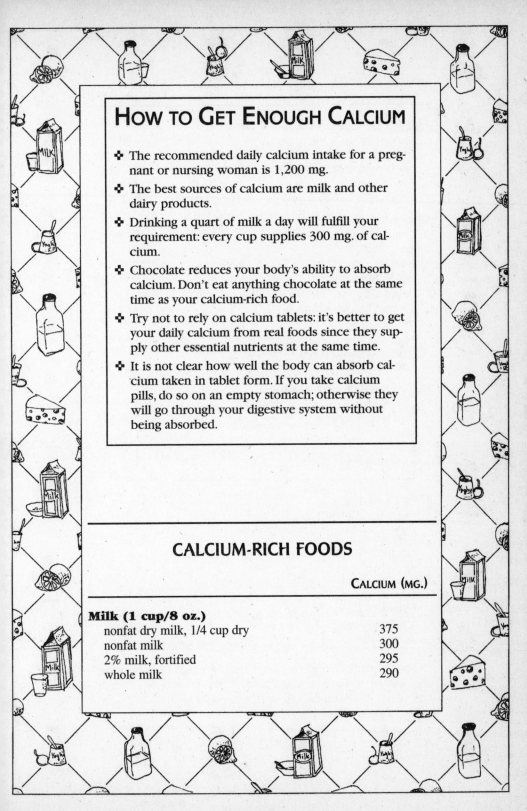

HOW TO GET ENOUGH CALCIUM

✤ The recommended daily calcium intake for a pregnant or nursing woman is 1,200 mg.

✤ The best sources of calcium are milk and other dairy products.

✤ Drinking a quart of milk a day will fulfill your requirement: every cup supplies 300 mg. of calcium.

✤ Chocolate reduces your body's ability to absorb calcium. Don't eat anything chocolate at the same time as your calcium-rich food.

✤ Try not to rely on calcium tablets: it's better to get your daily calcium from real foods since they supply other essential nutrients at the same time.

✤ It is not clear how well the body can absorb calcium taken in tablet form. If you take calcium pills, do so on an empty stomach; otherwise they will go through your digestive system without being absorbed.

CALCIUM-RICH FOODS

	CALCIUM (MG.)
Milk (1 cup/8 oz.)	
nonfat dry milk, 1/4 cup dry	375
nonfat milk	300
2% milk, fortified	295
whole milk	290

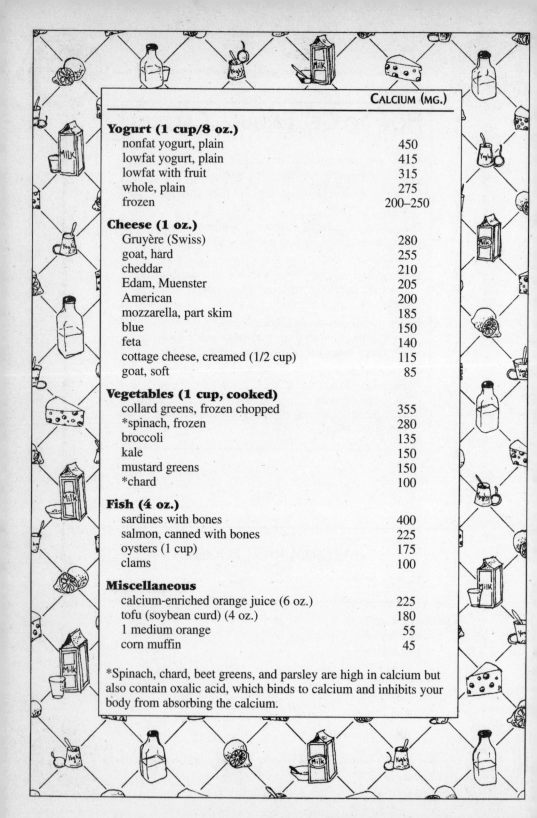

CALCIUM (MG.)

Yogurt (1 cup/8 oz.)

nonfat yogurt, plain	450
lowfat yogurt, plain	415
lowfat with fruit	315
whole, plain	275
frozen	200–250

Cheese (1 oz.)

Gruyère (Swiss)	280
goat, hard	255
cheddar	210
Edam, Muenster	205
American	200
mozzarella, part skim	185
blue	150
feta	140
cottage cheese, creamed (1/2 cup)	115
goat, soft	85

Vegetables (1 cup, cooked)

collard greens, frozen chopped	355
*spinach, frozen	280
broccoli	135
kale	150
mustard greens	150
*chard	100

Fish (4 oz.)

sardines with bones	400
salmon, canned with bones	225
oysters (1 cup)	175
clams	100

Miscellaneous

calcium-enriched orange juice (6 oz.)	225
tofu (soybean curd) (4 oz.)	180
1 medium orange	55
corn muffin	45

*Spinach, chard, beet greens, and parsley are high in calcium but also contain oxalic acid, which binds to calcium and inhibits your body from absorbing the calcium.

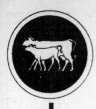
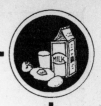

PROTEIN

* Protein foods are important for the development of your baby.
* You will probably need at least 75 grams every day.
* That is for a woman who's 5′2″ and 120 pounds—if there's more of you than that you'll need closer to 100 grams a day.

The best sources of protein
- MEAT
- FISH
- MILK
- CHEESE
- EGGS

* Vegetables have only a small amount of protein.
* Fruits have barely any protein.
* High-protein snacks include:
  - soynuts
  - peanut butter with wheat crackers
  - peanut butter with celery
  - cottage cheese with corn chips
  - whole-grain baked breads or cookies
  - nuts and seeds

Protein your body can use
* Our bodies can't fully use the protein in the food we eat.
* To choose foods that will help your baby grow big and healthy you need to know which protein your body can actually use.

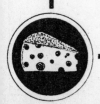
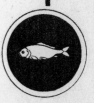

45

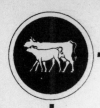
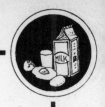

HIGH-PROTEIN FOODS

	Grams Protein	Usable Grams
Type of flour (1 cup)		
soybean, defatted	65	40
gluten	85	23
peanut, defatted	48	21
soybean, full fat	26	16
whole or cracked wheat	16	10
rye, dark	16	9
oatmeal, barley	11	7
cornmeal, whole ground	10	5
Meat and poultry		
turkey, 3 slices	31	22
pork chop, with fat	29	19
steak, 1/2 lb. without fat	25	17
hamburger, 1/4 lb.	26	17
chicken breast	23	15
lamb chop with fat	20	13
Fish (3 1/2 oz.)		
halibut	22	17
sardines, 3 canned in oil	21	14
swordfish, bass, shrimp	19	15
cod, Pacific herring, haddock	18	14
crab, northern lobster	17	14
squid, 3 sea scallops, sole	15	12
clams, 4 large or 8 small	14	11
oysters, 3	11	9
Dairy products (1 oz. or 1 sq. in.)		
cottage cheese (3 oz.), uncreamed	17	13
cottage cheese (3 oz.), creamed	14	11
milk, nonfat dry solids	10	8
Parmesan cheese	10	7
milk, 1 cup (any kind)	9	7
yogurt, nonfat, 1 cup	8	7
Swiss cheese	8	6
ricotta (1/4 cup), cheddar	7	5
ice cream	5	4

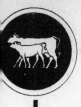

Legumes:
dried peas and beans
(1 cup cooked)

soybeans or soy grits	17	10
broad beans	13	6
peas, black-eyed peas, lentils	17	10
black beans, kidney beans	17	10
tofu (wet, 3 oz.)	8	5
navy, white, or pea beans; garbanzos	11	4

Grains and cereals

egg noodles (1 cup)	7	4
bulgur or cracked wheat (1/3 cup)	6	4
barley, millet (1/3 cup)	6	4
spaghetti, all pastas	5	3
oatmeal (1/3 cup)	4	3
rice, any kind	5	3
wheat germ (2 tbs.)	3	2
bread, 1 slice wheat or rye	2	1

Nuts and seeds (2 tbs.)

pine nuts (pignoli)	9	5
pumpkin/squash seeds	8	5
sunflower seeds (3 tbs.)	7	4
peanuts, peanut butter	8	3
cashews (15), pistachios (3 tbs.)	9	5
sesame seeds (3 tbs.), black walnuts	5	3

Vegetables (cooked weight)

lima beans (1/2 cup)	8	4
corn (1 ear), broccoli (3/4 cup)	4	2
collards (1/2 cup), mushrooms (12)	3	2
asparagus (6 spears)	3	2
artichoke, 1 large	6	2
cauliflower (1 cup), spinach (1/2 cup)	3	1.5
potato, medium baking	4	1

Nutritional additives

egg white, powdered (1/2 oz.)	11	9
Tiger's milk (1/4 cup)	8	6
brewer's yeast (1 tbs.)	4	2

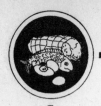
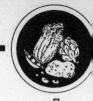

IRON

You should include iron-rich foods in your diet whenever possible, even though you can't be sure how much your body is actually absorbing.

Why you need extra iron

- Most women don't have enough iron stored in their bodies to meet the increased need during pregnancy.
- Your blood volume doubles when you're pregnant: iron is essential for the formation of healthy red blood cells.
- Your growing baby will take all the iron she or he needs from your body, no matter how low your iron supply may be.
- If you're deficient in iron you can become anemic, exhausted, and susceptible to infection.

HOW TO GET ENOUGH IRON

✤ It's hard to eat enough iron-rich foods to meet your body's new requirements.

✤ Even if you eat a lot of iron-rich foods your body can absorb only a small amount of the iron in them.

✤ Iron supplements (from 30 to 60 mg. a day) are recommended for all pregnant women. Talk to your doctor about your needs.

✤ Drinking tea or coffee with your food lowers the amount of iron your body can absorb.

✤ Ways to increase the absorption of iron:
  - High-acid foods (like yogurt and tomatoes) increase your body's ability to absorb iron from pills and food.
  - Foods high in vitamin C increase absorption.

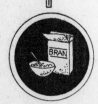
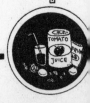

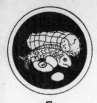

IRON-RICH FOODS

	MILLIGRAMS
Cereals (1 cup)	
40% bran flakes	11
raisin bran	9
cream of wheat	8
wheat germ (1/2 cup)	5
oatmeal	1.5
shredded wheat	1
Fish and meat (4 oz.)	
kidney	15
liver (chicken)	10
liver (beef)	9
clams	8
oysters	7
turkey	4.5
beef	4
sardines	3
lamb	2
pork or chicken	1
egg (1)	1
Fruit and juices (1 cup)	
apricots (dried)	8
raisins	3.5
prune juice	3
tomato juice	1.5
apple juice	1
dried figs (2), prunes (10)	1
Vegetables (1/2 cup cooked)	
beans, all kinds	2
artichoke (1)	2
peas, brussels sprouts	1.5
spinach, raw or cooked	1.5
Swiss chard	1
potato (white or sweet), raw tomato	.5
romaine lettuce (1 cup raw)	.5
Nuts (1/4 cup)	
almonds, cashews	1.5
walnuts	1

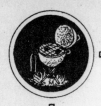
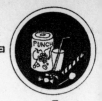

DANGERS IN FOODS

Beware of the barbecue

- Grilling meat or fish over hot charcoal, wood, or "bricks" can be dangerous.
    - ❧ Barbecuing produces carcinogens, which are substances that can cause cancer.
    - ❧ Carcinogens form when fat drips onto hot coals.
    - ❧ Carcinogens can also be formed when cooking at high temperatures by methods like frying or boiling.
- There are ways to grill and prevent carcinogens from forming. See below.
- Instead of grilling try roasting or baking.
- The safest methods of cooking are stewing, poaching, or microwaving.

LOW-RISK GRILLING

- ✤ Choose lean meat.
- ✤ Trim excess fat before grilling.
- ✤ Precook meat before barbecuing: boil it quickly or cook it in a microwave and pour off the juice.
- ✤ The meat juices contain the harmful substances: precooking destroys up to 90 percent of them.
- ✤ Cover the grill with aluminum foil, punching holes to let the fat drip out.
- ✤ Eat meat medium or medium rare, not well done. (This seems a contradiction of the advice to cook meat well to prevent toxoplasmosis, page 38.)
- ✤ More carcinogens are created the longer you cook on the grill.
- ✤ When barbecuing strike a balance between "bloody rare" and "well-done."
- ✤ Some foods like fish can be wrapped in foil to protect them.
- ✤ Keep a squirt bottle by the barbecue to dampen coals that flare up.
- ✤ The dangerous compounds form mainly on the outside of the food: after barbecuing try to remove the outer layer.

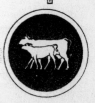

Food additives
- Many prepared foods and snacks contain additives.
- The less that's been done to food before you eat or cook it, the safer and more nutritious it is for you and your growing baby.
- Food additives have not been proven to be safe for your developing baby.

Artificial colors
- Snack foods and drinks are frequently colored with dyes.
- Avoid artificial colors in foods.
- As a rule of thumb, avoid products that are vividly false shades of orange, red, or purple.
- Look for foods that say "no artificial colors" on the package.

Hormones and antibiotics in red meat
- Antibiotics and growth hormones are often put in cattle feed.
- These substances remain in the meat you eat and may have an effect on your unborn child.
- Diethylstilbestrol (DES) is another drug given to cattle that accumulates in the animals' livers. Cattle cannot be fed DES for two weeks before slaughter but it's probably not worth the risk of eating liver.
- Buy meat from a market supplied by sources that don't use additives in their animal feed.
- There will be signs at meat counters declaring the food to be chemical-free.

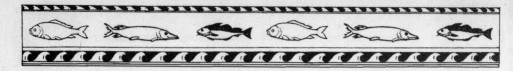

HAZARDS OF EATING FISH

Eating fish was once considered healthy but pollution and other problems mean there are now hazards to eating fish. The risk is even greater for pregnant women.

Buying fish
→ Be choosy about where you buy your fish.
→ Shops with high turnovers or that specialize in fish are your best bet.
→ Don't buy from a store where raw and cooked fish are displayed side by side: the bacteria from the raw can affect the cooked.
→ Don't buy fish piled high in open cases or under hot lights, which allow bacteria to grow faster.
→ Fish gills should be bright red or pink.
→ Fillets or steaks should have moist flesh with a translucent sheen, as if you can almost see inside.
→ Fish should not have a bad or fishy smell. A light, mild odor means freshness.

Things to avoid
- Discoloration
- Tears or other blemishes
- Brownish yellow stickiness
- Scale loss
- Red bruising

Preparing fish
→ Bring fish home from the store as quickly as possible and store in the coldest part of the refrigerator.
→ Bacteria multiply rapidly in fish if it's not stored at 32 degrees Fahrenheit or less. *Most home refrigerators are about 40 degrees.*
→ Fish is highly perishable and should be cooked within a day of buying.

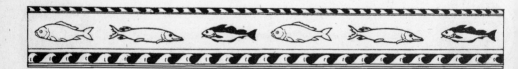

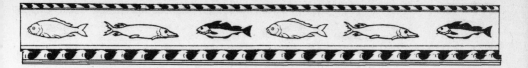

→ Wash your hands carefully after handling raw fish.
→ All utensils and surfaces the fish has touched should be thoroughly washed and rinsed with hot water.
→ Handle raw and cooked fish separately.
→ Cook fish and shellfish thoroughly, to an internal temperature of 140 degrees, or until it flakes easily.
→ Thaw frozen seafood in the refrigerator: *not* at room temperature and *not* under warm water.
→ As an extra precaution reheat "cooked, ready-to-eat shrimp" to destroy any bacteria that might be in them.

Fish to avoid

→ Forget the sushi bar: raw or barely cooked fish can harbor bacteria or parasites.
→ Do not eat raw clams or oysters: raw oysters have been singled out as having the highest health risk.
→ Raw shrimp are frequently contaminated with salmonella.
→ Frozen, "ready-to-eat" shrimp often have high levels of bacterial contamination.
→ Avoid fish from "hot spots":
  ❧ Water with high levels of chemical contaminants can affect the fish, which can cause birth defects.
  ❧ The Great Lakes, Santa Monica Bay, Puget Sound, and Chesapeake Bay are examples of hot spots.
  ❧ Women of childbearing age in the Great Lakes region have been cautioned to avoid all fish from that area.

Shellfish safety

→ Live shellfish should be refrigerated, not held in water.
→ Scallops should be translucent; they should not be opaque even at the edges.
→ The fact that live crabs and lobsters are in a tank does not guarantee quality. Ask how long they've been in there.
→ Whole cracked crabs should be displayed in or on ice.
→ Any bivalve—clam, oyster, mussel, scallop—with an open shell is dead and not edible.

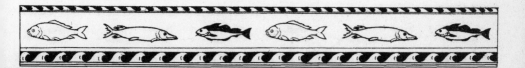

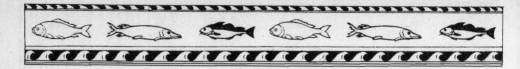

Cautions about specific fish

→ *Swordfish* often has high levels of methyl mercury, which is considered a "reproductive toxin" and is to be avoided by any woman even contemplating pregnancy.

→ *Tuna and mahimahi* also contain mercury, although at lower levels than swordfish.

→ *Whitefish, East Coast salmon, and shark* may have high levels of PCBs, which are harmful to the fetus.

→ *"Recreationally caught"* fish often come from waters of suspect quality and tend to be mishandled after catching.

Safest fish to eat

→ Flounder and sole are the only two fresh fish commonly found virtually free of pollutants.

→ Experts say salmon is one of the most trouble-free fresh fish.

→ Canned tuna, salmon, and other canned fish are very safe.

→ Processed frozen products like fish sticks, breaded fillets, and nuggets made from white-fleshed fish such as cod, haddock, and pollock are safe if kept frozen.

→ Farmed fish like catfish, trout, and salmon have a good record for being free from disease.

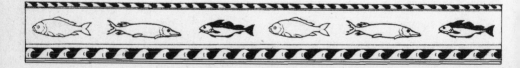

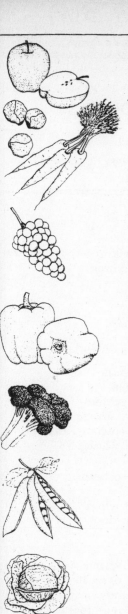

VEGETARIAN PREGNANCY

Are you getting enough protein?

- A vegetarian dish can be perfectly healthy during pregnancy as long as you make sure you're getting enough protein. The quality and amount of protein you eat should be your main concerns.
- Without enough protein you are more prone to complications in labor.
- Protein needs can be met differently if you are a "vegan" (a complete vegetarian, who eats no animal products) or a "lacto-vegetarian," who eats dairy products.
- See the section on protein, pages 45–47.

Why is protein so important to vegetarians?

- Most plant foods (unlike animal foods) don't have all the essential amino acids in the necessary amounts.
- If an amino acid is missing from a protein food it is "incomplete" and your body cannot use it . . . but if you eat the correct combination of several plant foods at the same meal it transforms the foods into complete proteins that your body can then fully utilize.
- All pregnant vegetarians can benefit from *Diet for a Small Planet* by Frances Moore Lappé, which will help you combine foods to their best benefit. The following chart was adapted from that book to give you easy reference.
- If you eat foods in the combinations listed on the following chart, the missing amino acids will be completed. Keep this chart handy throughout your pregnancy so you can eat complete proteins.

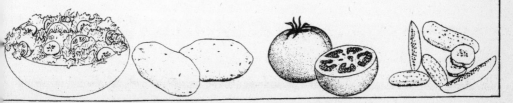

COMPLEMENTARY PLANT PROTEIN SOURCES

Food	Amino Acids Deficient	Complementary Protein
Grains	Isoleucine Lysine	rice + legumes corn + legumes wheat + legumes wheat + peanut + milk wheat + sesame + soybean rice + sesame rice + brewer's yeast
Legumes	Tryptophan Methionine	legumes + rice beans + wheat beans + corn soybeans + rice + wheat soybeans + corn + milk soybeans + wheat + sesame soybeans + peanuts + sesame soybeans + peanuts + wheat + rice soybeans + sesame + wheat
Nuts and seeds	Isoleucine Lysine	peanuts + sesame + soybeans sesame + beans sesame + soybeans + wheat peanuts + sunflower seeds
Vegetables	Isoleucine Methionine	lima beans green peas brussels sprouts + sesame seeds or Brazil nuts or mushrooms cauliflower broccoli greens + millet or converted rice

How to eat enough protein

→ Even eggs and milk are not absolute requirements for getting enough protein, but a vegetarian must constantly pay attention to the ingredients of her diet to insure enough protein.

→ *If you are a complete vegetarian* you can get sufficient protein if you eat (in addition to your grains and vegetables) the following combinations every day:

    • 1 cup soybeans plus 12 oz. soymilk or soy yogurt

OR

    • 1/2 lb. tofu plus a pint soymilk or soy yogurt

OR

    • 1 qt. soymilk or soy yogurt plus 1/2 cup soybeans

OR

    • 1 cup hydrated TVP (texturized vegetable protein) plus 1 cup soymilk or soy yogurt

→ *If you are a lacto-vegetarian* (you eat dairy products), then in addition to your vegetables and grains, you can get enough protein by eating daily:

    • 2 cups cottage cheese

OR

    • 1 qt. skim milk, low-fat yogurt or buttermilk *plus* 1/2 cup cottage cheese

→ Keep high-protein snacks handy: soynuts, peanut butter on wheat crackers or celery, cottage cheese with corn chips.

→ Many vegetarian diets are not nutritionally sound and don't supply enough protein for general health . . . much less pregnancy. Please make an extra effort to protect yourself and your baby by taking in lots of high quality protein.

SUPPLEMENTS FOR THE NONLACTO-VEGETARIAN

If you don't include milk in your vegetarian diet then you *must* have the following supplements every day:

    ✦ 12 mg. calcium

    ✦ 400 I.U. vitamin D

    ✦ 4 mg. vitamin B_{12}

    ✦ 1.5 mg. riboflavin

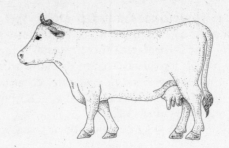

COW'S MILK COMPARED TO SOYBEAN

	Calcium (mg.)	Calories	Protein (gm.)	Fat (gm.)	Iron (mg.)
Whole milk (8 oz.)	290	160	8	8	0.1
Soybean milk	47	75	8	3	2.5
Tofu (Soybean curd) (4 oz.)	155	86	9.5	5	2.5

VEGETARIAN DAILY FOOD PYRAMID

The following food pyramid shows you the building blocks you need as a vegetarian for a healthy pregnancy. Vegans (those vegetarians who don't eat eggs or dairy products) need to pay special attention to the top of the pyramid. All vegetarians should make an effort to "build" one of these complete food pyramids every day, with the recommended number of servings from each level of the pyramid.

Base of the pyramid (6 to 10 servings)
* Bread
* Cereals
* Pasta
* Rice
* Corn
* Potatoes
* Green peas

Two sides of the second level
* Vegetables (2 to 4 servings)
* Fruits (2 to 4 servings)

Two sides of the upper level
* Milk and milk substitutes (2 to 4)
* Protein (2 to 4)

Top of the pyramid (for Vegans)
* Vegetable oil (2 tablespoons)
* Blackstrap molasses (1 tablespoon)
* Brewer's yeast (1 tablespoon)

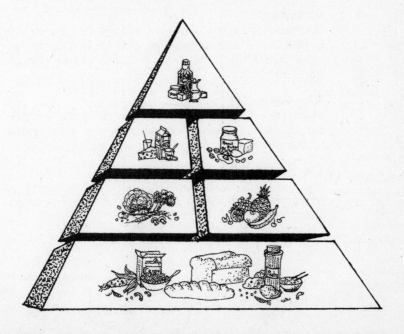

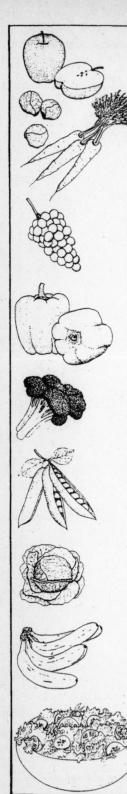

POSSIBLE DEFICIENCIES
FOR VEGETARIANS

Iodine
Use iodized salt. Sea salt does not supply iodine, which your thyroid gland needs during the extra stress of pregnancy.

Iron
You should probably have your blood tested throughout pregnancy to check your iron level since vegetarian diets usually don't supply enough. Depending on the results you should take one 5-grain tablet three times a day. Take 100 mg. vitamin C each time to help your body absorb the iron. Take the iron tablet with meals so it's easier on your stomach.

Calcium
Dairy products are the source for calcium. Some plant foods supply calcium but your body can't utilize it very well. If you're not a lacto-vegetarian you need 1 gram a day for the second half of your pregnancy and during nursing. Calcium gluconate is the best form, in two 500 mg. tablets.

Vitamin D
Fortified cow's milk or soymilk contains D. If those are not in your diet you need to supplement vitamin D. (But no more than 400 I.U. daily—see "Vitamins Can Be Dangerous," page 22.)

Riboflavin
Milk is the best source. A nonlacto-vegetarian may not have enough in her system because there are only limited amounts in whole grains, legumes, nuts, and vegetables.

Vitamin B$_{12}$
Milk and animal foods supply this nutrient. A deficiency of B$_{12}$ can cause you serious complications so be sure to get a supplement if you don't drink milk.

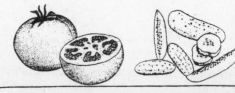

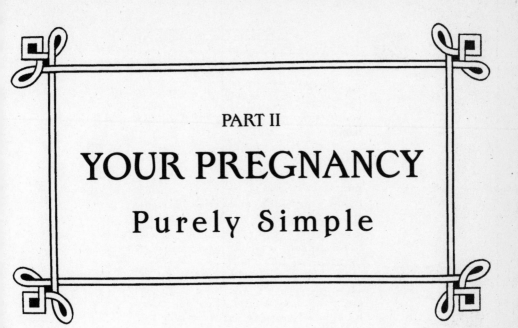

PART II

YOUR PREGNANCY

Purely Simple

3.
Your Growing Baby
Week by Week

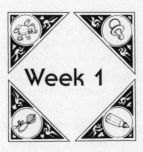

Week 1

* Once the egg and sperm unite, the cells begin dividing. They travel along your fallopian tube until they reach your uterus, around the fourth day after fertilization.
* The cells then multiply into the blastocyst: a round, solid, growing mass of about one hundred cells.
    * The outer layer of the blastocyst becomes the placenta.
    * The inner layer becomes what is known as the embryo.

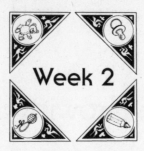

Week 2

* In the second week there are 150 cells that make up the embryo.
* The cells are divided into three layers of tissue that will develop separately:
    * The inside layer becomes the breathing and digestive organs.
    * The middle layer is going to develop into bones, cartilage, muscles, the circulatory system, kidneys, and sex organs.
    * The outside layer becomes your baby's skin and nerves.
* During this second week the embryo floats freely in your uterus, nourished by secretions from the uterine lining.

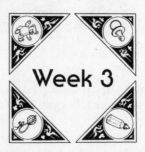

Week 3

* By the end of the third week the embryo begins to attach to the wall of your uterus.
* The preliminary tissues become a tubular, folded structure with the beginnings of a heart, brain, and spinal cord.
* The outer cells surrounding the embryo spread out like roots into your uterine lining.
* The deepest cells form the basis of what will become the placenta, which will nourish the baby.
* Other cells are developing into the amniotic sac, which will surround the placenta.

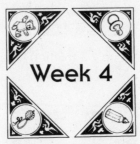

Week 4

(End of 1st Month)

* By the end of the fourth week the minuscule embryo has formed into the shape of a tadpole.
* The rudimentary beginnings of arms occur on the twenty-sixth day.
* On the twenty-eighth day the basic beginnings of legs develop. The legs will be slower in development than the arms.
* The embryo is less than one tenth of an inch long, or smaller than a grain of rice. It would be barely visible to your naked eye.

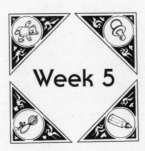

Week 5

* By the end of the fifth week the foundation has been laid for what will be your baby's brain, spinal cord, and nervous system.
* Groups of tissue are developing that will later become your baby's spine, ribs, and abdominal muscles.
* Your baby's backbone is also forming, with five to eight vertebrae laid down.
* The neural tube, which is the first step in the development of the central nervous system, forms.
    * One end of this will become your baby's brain.
    * The other end becomes the spinal cord.

* A tubular, *S*-shaped heart is beginning to beat. This beating heart is located on the outside of the body, not yet inside the chest cavity.
* The developing baby is only a fraction of an inch long.

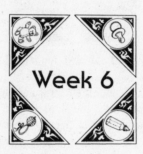

Week 6

* At the beginning of the sixth week the head is starting to form. There is the beginning of a brain.
* There are depressions beneath the skin where the eyes and ears will later appear.
* A two-chamber heart is forming. This will eventually become a four-chamber organ.
* The baby's intestinal tract is forming. This starts from the mouth cavity downward, although the mouth cannot yet open.
* The stalk connecting the embryo to the placenta begins to grow into the umbilical cord, with blood vessels inside it through which you will nourish your growing child.
* By the end of this week the entire backbone has been laid down and the spinal canal is closed over. However, the lower part of the back is still undeveloped.
* The baby grows in a curved sea horse shape because the blocks of tissue in the back of the embryo grow more quickly than those in front.
* At the corners of the body there are tiny limb buds (which first appeared in the fourth week) that will later become the arms and legs. The germ cells, which will later become either ovaries or testes, have appeared.
* By the end of this week your baby will be one fourth of an inch long.

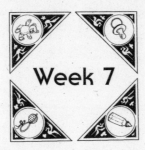

Week 7

* Nerves and muscles work together for the first time now.
* The baby has reflexes and makes spontaneous movements (although you probably won't feel these until the sixteenth to twenty-sixth weeks).
* The chest and abdomen are completely formed and the lung buds are appearing.
* The heart is now inside the body. The heart is still a simple structure but it has developed four chambers beating with enough strength to circulate blood cells through the blood vessels.
* By the end of this week your baby's brain and spinal cord will be almost complete.
* During this week the embryo becomes a primitive small-scale baby with a lumpy head that is bent forward on the chest.
* The baby's mouth can open, with lips and a tongue visible.
* The face looks more human, with eyes perceptible through closed lids and openings for the nostrils.
* Shell-like external ears are developing, although they don't yet protrude.
    * This is an important week for the growth of your baby's inner ear.
    * The middle part of the ear, which is responsible for balance as well as hearing, develops.
* The limb buds are growing rapidly and there is a paddle shape to what will be arms and legs.
* The hands have the beginnings of fingers and thumbs. The toes are stubby but the big toes have appeared.
* The baby's arms are as long as this exclamation point (!).
* The baby's overall length is about half an inch, or roughly the size of your thumbnail, by the end of the seventh week.

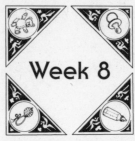

Week 8

(End of 2nd Month)

* In this week—actually, on the forty-seventh day of your pregnancy—the first true bone cells begin to replace cartilage.
* This is the baby's official transition from embryo to fetus.
* The bones of the arms and legs start to harden and elongate.
* Critical joines like the knee, hips, shoulders, and elbows are forming.
* Toes and fingers are more pronounced, although they are joined by webs of skin.
* By the end of this week the baby's physical structure is complete with a skeleton mode of cartilage that will gradually be replaced by bone cells.
* The body has a fishlike shape and the head is disproportionately large.
* The face and jaw are fully formed, with the teeth and facial muscles still developing.
* The eyes are covered by skin that will eventually split to form the eyelids.
* The heart is now pumping forcefully with a regular rhythm. Blood vessels are visible through the transparent skin.
* All the major organs—heart, brain, lungs, kidneys, liver, and intestines—are in place, although not yet fully developed.
* The clitoris or penis begins to appear. The ovaries or testicles are taking form; however, at this point you couldn't tell just by looking whether it's a girl or a boy.
* By the end of this second month the baby weighs about one third of an ounce (less than an aspirin tablet) and is a little more than one inch long.

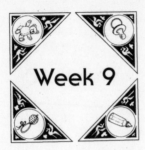

Week 9

* Physical refinements are taking place and the baby's face is becoming quite human except for the jaws, which aren't fully developed.
* During these seven days the baby will start to open the mouth.
    * Once the upper and lower jaws fuse at the sides the baby will be able to suck and chew.
    * The palate to form the roof of the mouth is closing.
* Taste buds and the glands that produce saliva appear; the vocal cords are developing.
* Tooth buds for the baby teeth are present.
* The eyes, which were at the sides of the head, are moving to the front. Their development is complete, although they still have a membrane eyelid.
* A nose has appeared.
* The fastest growth this week is in the limbs, hands, and feet. Fingers and toes are becoming defined and nail beds are forming for eventual nails.
* The chest cavity becomes separated from the abdominal cavity by a band of muscle that will later develop into the diaphragm, a muscle that plays an important part in breathing.
* The heart has completed forming four chambers and is beating 117 to 157 beats per minute.
* The baby is just over an inch in length this week. The hands are now about as big (one fourth of an inch) as the whole embryo was a month ago.

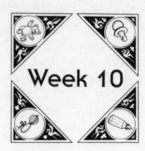

Week 10

* The baby's brain has developed quickly in the past month so that the head is still large in proportion to the body.
* This week marks the final development of the ears: the inner portion is complete and the external parts are beginning to grow.
* The stomach and intestines have formed in the abdomen, and the muscle wall of the intestinal tract is developing.
* The kidneys are moving into their permanent positions and will have developed by the end of this month.
* The lungs are growing inside the chest cavity.
* The major blood vessels are assuming their final form.
* The umbilical cord has fully formed and blood is circulating through it.
* By this week the baby has grown to just under one and a half inches.

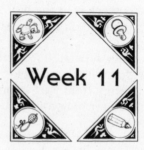

Week 11

* The baby is now able to swallow, and the cycle of circulation starts.
* The kidneys have formed and the urinary system is operating: the baby swallows amniotic fluid and urinates it back into the amniotic fluid in which he floats.

* All your baby's essential organs will have formed by the end of this week and most of them are beginning to function. From this point the organs will simply continue to grow.
  * The liver is now producing bile.
  * Your baby's heart is pumping blood to all parts of the body.
  * Blood is also being pumped through the umbilical cord to what is going to become the placenta.
* Your baby is now clearly recognizable as a tiny human with a face that's becoming more rounded.
* The back of the head has enlarged, which puts the eyes in a more natural position than before; the ears have a flatter shape and are continuing to develop.
* The limbs are still short and skinny but the ankles and wrists have formed and the elbows and knees are taking shape.
* The toes and fingers are now clearly separated and developed.
* The baby's length is now approximately two inches.

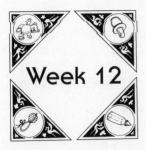

Week 12

(End of 3rd Month)

* With a signal from the brain, the baby's muscles now respond and she or he kicks. However, all movements reflex from the spinal cord since the brain is not yet sufficiently organized to control them (and it won't be until after birth).
* The baby is becoming active but unless you are very slender it is rare to feel the movement yet.
* She can make stepping movements and even curl her toes.
* The brain and muscles coordinate so that the arms bend and can rotate at the wrist and elbow.
* The fingers close so that the baby can form a tight fist or unclench it.
* The ears are completely formed.

* He can make facial expressions like pressing the lips together and frowning.
* He is already using the muscles required for breathing after birth.
* The female external vulva and male penis have gradually been molded during the second and third months. The male scrotum appears during the twelfth week, although it is still difficult to distinguish the baby's sex at this point.
* This week the umbilical cord starts to circulate blood between the baby and the group of membranes attached to the wall of your uterus. Your baby's body has begun to depend on these membranes for nourishment: the placenta begins to function this week.
* By the end of the third month the baby weighs a little more than half an ounce.

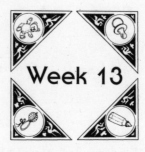

Week 13

* By the end of this week your baby is properly formed and fills the uterine cavity.
* The neck is now fully developed, allowing the head to move freely on the body.
* The face is formed, with the mouth, nose, and external ears completely developed.
* By the end of this week your baby is three inches long and weighs about one ounce.

A WORD ABOUT THE PLACENTA

✤ The placenta is an organ created by your body to nourish your baby and excrete his waste products.

✤ The placenta looks like a large, roundish liver. It is one inch thick and measures about eight inches in diameter.

✤ It was fully formed by last week and will be fully operational by next week.

✤ The placenta is attached on one side to your uterus and on the other side to the baby's umbilical cord.

✤ It is the baby's lifeline to you: your blood, carrying oxygen and nutrients, reaches the baby through a fine membrane into the placenta.

✤ The placenta functions like a sieve, passing oxygen, food, and protective antibodies from you to your baby (although harmful elements can also filter through).

✤ The baby gets rid of waste products by filtering them through the placenta into your bloodstream, allowing you to excrete them.

✤ The blood from which the baby has already taken oxygen comes back through an artery in the umbilical cord into the placenta.

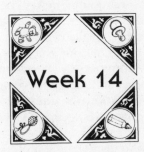

Week 14

* This week marks the beginning of the second trimester of your pregnancy, the time when your baby does most of her growing and when her organs mature.
* The baby's heart is beating strongly (her heartbeat is almost twice as fast as yours), and you may be able to hear it in the doctor's office.

* Her nervous system has begun to function and her muscles respond to stimulation from her brain.
* Her arms continue their development of specialized functions and can grasp, curl, and make fists.
* Her movements are more vigorous but you probably don't feel them yet.
* The baby develops her muscles by exercising energetically inside you, which she does with ease, floating in the amniotic fluid.
* During this past week your baby has more than doubled in weight. She now weighs over two ounces and measures around four inches in length.

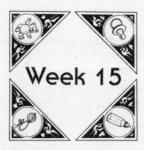

Week 15

* Your baby is able to hear by now because the three tiny bones of his middle ear are the first of his bones to harden.
    * From now on *you* are what he will be listening to! Liquid is a good sound conductor, so through the amniotic fluid the baby can hear your heart beating, your stomach rumbling, and the sound of your voice.
    * Certain sounds from outside the womb can also reach him.
    * His brain is not yet sufficiently developed, however, to process the information: the auditory centers in the brain (which decipher sounds received) have not yet fully formed.
* Your baby has begun to grow hair sometime in the past week: by now there's a little fluff on his head and he has eyebrows along with white eyelashes.
* The *lanugo* starts to grow:
    * A fine, downy hair begins to appear all over your baby's face and body. This hair keeps his temperature constant.

❦ Most of this hair will disappear before he is born.

❦ Whatever is left will fall out soon after birth.

* The baby now measures somewhat more than five inches and weighs roughly three and a half ounces.

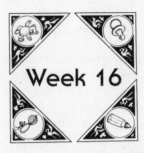

Week 16

(End of 4th Month)

* By the end of the fourth month the baby will suck if her lips are stroked.
    ❦ If a bitter substance like iodine is introduced into the amniotic fluid she will grimace and stop swallowing.
    ❦ If a sweetener is introduced she usually drinks twice as quickly.
* If a bright light is shined on your abdomen the baby will gradually move her hands up to shield her eyes.
* In these weeks the baby is moving actively and can even turn somersaults, although if this is your first child you probably won't feel these movements.
* At sixteen weeks some babies may begin to suck their thumb, which helps develop coordination and has a soothing effect.
* At this point your baby can yawn, stretch, and make facial expressions.
* She can also swallow and may get hiccups.
* Her eyes are large, spaced wide apart, and closed.
* During the fourth month the baby grows so much she quadruples her weight and doubles her height. She now weighs about seven ounces and is six inches long.

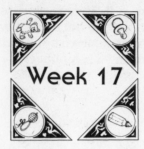

Week 17

* Your baby's skin is developing and is transparent. It appears red because the blood vessels are visible through it.
* The baby's skin has begun to develop *vernix,* a white protective coating like cream cheese.
* The hair on his head, eyebrows, and eyelashes is filling out.
* Hard nails form on the nail beds, with the toenails developing a bit later than the fingernails.
* Both sexes develop nipples and underlying mammary glands.
* The external genital organs have now developed sufficiently for your baby's sex to be detected by ultrasound.
* Your baby measures a little more than seven inches in length and now weighs more than the placenta does.

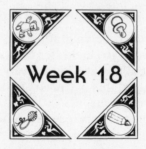

Week 18

* The baby can now hear sounds outside your body:
    * If a loud sound is made next to you the unborn baby will raise his hands and cover his ears.
    * Very loud sounds have been known to startle the baby enough to make him jump inside you.
* His limbs are fully developed and all his joints are able to move. He's testing his reflexes by kicking and punching with well-formed arms and legs.
* He is moving around much of the time. It's during this week that

you may feel his gyration for the first time. He can twist, turn, and wiggle inside you (and may practice when you least expect it!).

* The baby's muscles are now almost fully developed, including the muscles in his chest, which are beginning to make movements similar to those that he will use for respiration later on.
* Tiny air sacs, known as *alveoli,* are forming inside his developing lungs. He'll need these later in order to breathe.
* Your baby measures about eight inches long this week.

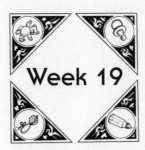

Week 19

* If you haven't felt the baby yet, you'll probably perceive the baby's movements this week.
* Buds for permanent teeth begin forming behind those that have already developed for her baby teeth.
* In some babies it is only during this week that they begin to grow hair and eyebrows and white eyelashes appear.
* Your baby now measures about nine inches long.

THE AMNIOTIC FLUID

✤ It is filled with salts and other nutrients that the baby absorbs through her skin, as she has been doing throughout your pregnancy.

✤ This fluid is always fresh because it's constantly being produced by your body. It is completely replenished every six hours.

✤ At this stage in development your baby is drinking quite a lot of amniotic fluid.

✤ Her stomach begins to secrete gastric juices, enabling her body to absorb those liquids.

✤ After the fluid is absorbed, her kidneys filter the fluid and excrete it back into the amniotic sac.

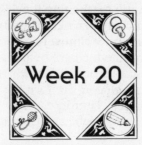

Week 20

(End of 5th Month)

* The baby's muscles are getting stronger every week. If you haven't felt them before, you can certainly feel his active movements now.
* His legs are now in proportion with the rest of his body and his movements are becoming increasingly sophisticated. The baby's kicking, punching, and tumbling will be a pretty constant part of your life for the next twenty weeks of pregnancy!
* Your baby is growing rapidly and has reached about ten inches in length. This is half of what he'll probably measure at birth. This rapid growth will soon slow down.
* By the end of this month, the baby weighs about twelve ounces.

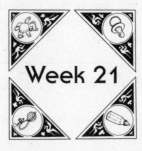

Week 21

* In the past few weeks, *vernix* (a white, greasy substance) has been forming on your baby's delicate, newly formed skin.
    * Vernix protects her from the liquid environment she has to live in all these months.
    * From this point in your pregnancy the vernix serves to protect the baby's skin from the increasing concentration of her urine in the amniotic fluid.
    * By the time your baby is ready to be born most of the vernix will have dissolved.

Ⱥ Some vernix will still be there to lubricate your baby's journey down the birth canal during labor and delivery.

* Your baby has now reached about eleven inches and weighs just under a pound.

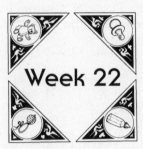

Week 22

* The baby's body has started to produce white blood cells. These are essential in order for her to be able to combat disease and infection.
* If your baby is a girl her internal organs of reproduction have formed by now.
* The baby is moving vigorously.
* You may notice that she responds to your touch or to sounds that reach her.
* If you haven't been aware of it before, you may feel a jerking motion inside you that is the baby having hiccups.
* By this week your baby's tongue is fully developed.
* Your baby has grown to about twelve inches long and weighs about one pound.

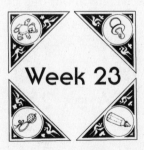

Week 23

* Until now the baby's skin has been transparent, with the blood vessels visible through it; now it becomes opaque. His skin is extremely wrinkled, with loose folds, almost as though he hasn't

"grown into it." This is because there aren't yet any fat deposits underneath his skin.
* Creases have begun to appear on his fingertips and the palms of his hands.
* By next week his fingerprints and toe prints will be visible.
* You can hear the baby's heartbeat through a stethoscope. Your husband may be able to hear the baby's heart by putting his ear directly against your stomach.

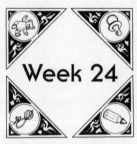

Week 24

(End of 6th Month)

* By this week the baby's hearing system is perfectly developed:
    * The organs of balance located in the inner ear have developed to the full dimensions they'll have for life.
    * Because water is a better sound conductor than air the baby in utero can hear, although with distortions. As your baby reacts to sound, her pulse rate increases.
    * She'll move in rhythm to music she hears.
* By the end of the baby's sixth month in your uterus she is thirteen inches long and weighs about one pound two ounces.

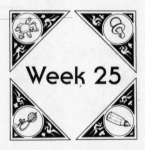

Week 25

* The baby's hands are active now and his muscular coordination has developed so that he's able to get his thumb into his mouth.

Thumb sucking calms the baby and strengthens jaw and cheek muscles.

* Although he's probably been hiccuping for some time, by this week he has a new skill: now he can cry!
* Your baby's bone centers are beginning to harden.
* At this point in your pregnancy his growth is slow and steady.
* The baby's body is fattening up and growing at a faster pace than his head, which until now has been disproportionately large.
* The baby's body is getting long and thin, with fat deposits building up under the skin.
* In the last week your baby has grown about half an inch and added some weight.
* He now measures fourteen inches and weighs around one pound four onces.

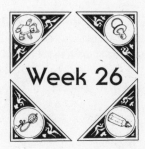

Week 26

* Recordings of the baby's brain waves at the beginning of the last trimester show that the baby has rapid eye movement (REM) sleep. In adults, REM sleep is associated with dreaming. This means that your unborn baby may be dreaming now.
* The branches of your baby's lungs (the bronchi) are developing.
    * His lungs won't be fully formed until after he's born.
    * If your baby was born prematurely now, however, there's a good chance his lungs would be able to function.
* The placenta's usefulness begins to diminish during this month.
* The amount of amniotic fluid decreases as the baby gets bigger.

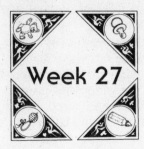

Week 27

* The membranes that covered your baby's eyes separate this week and her eyelids begin to part. She can open her eyes and look around for the first time. It isn't always dark inside your uterus: bright sunlight or artificial light can filter through the uterine wall.
* At this stage of development a baby's eyes are almost blue: the true eye color will generally not fully develop until a few months after birth.
* She now has fully developed eyebrows and delicate eyelashes.
* Your baby weighs about two pounds. However, her length has not changed much in the last two weeks: she's still about fourteen inches long.

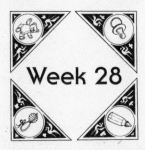

Week 28

(End of 7th Month)

* If your baby was born prematurely now, he has matured enough to be able to live independently.
* His lungs, which are essential for living outside the womb, are reaching maturity. (But if he was premature he might need medical help to breathe and maintain his body temperature.)

* By this twenty-eighth week of pregnancy a boy's testicles have descended into his scrotum.
* The baby has put on more than a pound in this month, for a total weight of about two pounds four ounces. His length has reached fifteen inches.

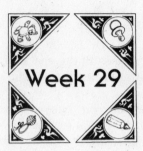

Week 29

* The baby can hear even more by this stage:
    * Previously he could mainly hear vibrations, but now the nerve endings in his ears are connected that enable him to hear sounds.
    * There are indications that some babies' hearing starts to develop earlier, but by now most babies can definitely hear distinct sounds.
    * Your baby can hear your voice now, which researchers know because his heart rate increases when his mother or father speaks.
    * This means your baby can also hear music, although it has to be played quite loudly since his ears are plugged by water and vernix.
    * After he's born, if the baby hears music you played before birth he may show he recognizes it by becoming less active while he listens.
* Your baby is gaining about seven ounces a week and now weighs about two pounds eleven ounces. His weekly growth in length is under half an inch.
* By this week he measures just a little more than fifteen inches.

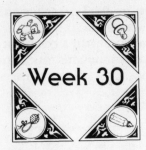

Week 30

* Your baby now fills almost all the space in your uterus.
* She may be lying with her head up or she may still have room to do somersaults.
* At any time from now on your baby will probably feel more comfortable when her head is settled down in your bony pelvis.
* Your baby's brain is growing rapidly and she's practicing opening her eyes and breathing.
* She weighs about three pounds two ounces this week.

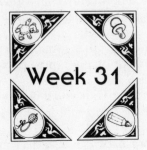

Week 31

* Your baby begins to move less inside you as she runs out of room. She's probably lying in a curled-up position, with her knees bent, her chin resting on her chest, and her arms and legs crossed.
* If she hasn't turned into a head-down position by this week, she will be likely to do so in the next seven days. Most babies turn into a vertex position to be born headfirst.
* If she doesn't turn, your doctor or midwife may try to turn the baby around by manipulating her from the outside.

* During this week the air sacs inside the baby's lungs become lined with a layer of cells that produce a liquid called *surfactant.* This material prevents the air sacs from collapsing when your baby first begins to breathe after birth.
* This week your baby measures just under sixteen inches and weighs about three pounds nine ounces.

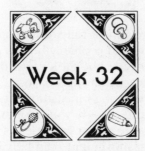

Week 32

(End of 8th Month)

* The baby is now likely to have settled into a vertex position, where he will stay until birth.
* Smaller babies with more room to move can bounce between vertex and breech (bottom-down) positions for several more weeks.
* You will know if your baby has turned into the head-down position because instead of the baby's head pressing against your ribs, you'll feel his feet kicking against your rib cage.
* The baby's elbows and knees may be more visible as they press against the uterine wall.
* Growth, especially of the brain, is great at this time.
* As your baby grows plumper the wrinkles in his skin fill out and he appears smoother.
* Both the lanugo and vernix that cover his skin begin to disappear around this time.
* By the end of the eighth month the baby weighs about four pounds, although he probably doesn't grow significantly in length this week.

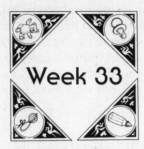

Week 33

* Your baby's lungs are almost fully developed, although if she was born now she would probably be placed in an incubator.
* She's still on the thin side but she's perfectly formed, with the proportions you'll see when she's born.
* She still doesn't have enough insulating fat deposits underneath her skin to keep warm outside your womb.
* You may be more aware of her activities as she takes up more room inside you. Her movements can be vigorous at this point and may cause you discomfort, especially if her feet get caught under your ribs.
* Your baby now weighs about four pounds seven ounces and measures more than one foot four inches.

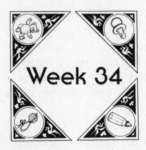

Week 34

* Growth, especially of the brain, has been enormous in the past few weeks.
* Most of the baby's systems are well developed, although her lungs may still be immature.
* She's probably trying to practice breathing using her lungs. However, since no air is available she swallows amniotic fluid into her windpipe, which can give her frequent hiccups.
* The baby's eyes are usually slate blue in color and she is practicing blinking.

* Her hair has been growing and can be as much as two inches long by this week.
* Your baby responds to familiar voices.
* By this week your baby weighs about four pounds fourteen ounces.

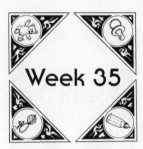

Week 35

* Your baby is getting rounder day by day, losing his wrinkled appearance as he plumps up.
* Between this week and when he is born he will continuously accumulate fat deposits beneath his skin.
* His skin is losing its redness and becomes pinker each day.
* Your baby weighs five pounds five ounces and is just under one foot five inches.

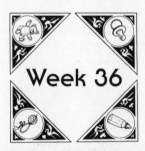

Week 36

(End of 9th Month)

* By now the baby is almost ready for birth. If he was born at this point, he would be premature but he would do well.
* In this last trimester of your pregnancy, the baby has received antibodies from you. He gets natural protection from whatever illnesses you've had, from measles to the common cold, or any diseases you've been immunized against, like polio or smallpox.

* The baby's rate of growth is slowing down, although this is the time when he needs to get more plump in preparation for life on the outside.
* Fat cells are being deposited under the baby's skin every day.
* During this month your baby has gained two pounds: he weighs five pounds twelve ounces and his length is one foot six inches.

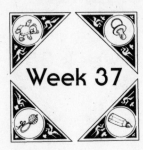

Week 37

* The baby's toenails and fingernails have grown to the tips of her toes and fingers.
* Her muscles have grown strong from vigorous motions of her arms and legs.
* She continues to practice the movements of her lungs she will need to breathe outside your body.
* All your baby's organs are now almost fully mature; only her lungs need a little longer to complete their development.
* If your baby is in a vertex position her head has probably dropped into your pelvis by this week.

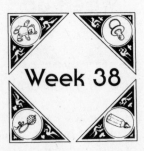

Week 38

* The baby's reflexes have become coordinated so that he can blink and close his eyes, turn his head, grasp firmly, and respond to sounds, light, and touch.

* He can differentiate between light and dark. He can see more if there is direct sunlight (or another source of bright light) shining directly on your stomach.
* The fine lanugo hair covering his body has been falling out. This process speeds up this week, although some hair may remain on his shoulders, in the folds of his skin, and maybe even on the back of his ears. Whatever lanugo is left when he's born will fall out in the early postpartum days.

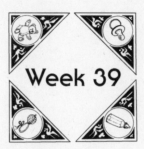

Week 39

* Your baby is now ready to be born.
* She's become plump enough by now, with the layer of fat that's been building up under her skin, to be able to regulate her body temperature after birth.
* Her skin is soft and smooth and her body has filled out.
* She may weigh anywhere from six to eleven pounds by the end of this week.
* Any time now you're going to be a *mother*!

4.
Moans and Groans of Pregnancy

Misery loves company! If it makes you feel any better, you're not alone: most pregnant women have at least some of the aches and pains that follow. This section is alphabetical and covers all the possible annoyances of being pregnant along with most of the known remedies.

ABDOMINAL PAIN

Signs and symptoms
- Most pregnant women experience abdominal pain. It's probably caused by the stretching of muscles and ligaments that support the uterus.
- It may be in the form of cramps or sharp, stabbing pains.
- It can be brief or last for several hours.

Helpful hints
→ If the pain is intermittent and not persistent—and you have no fever, bleeding, or unusual symptoms—there's no need to worry.
→ Sitting or lying in a comfortable position should help.
→ Always remember to mention the pain at your next visit to the doctor.

ALLERGIES

Causes and symptoms
- Pregnancy is a major stress on your body that can aggravate existing conditions or cause some women to develop allergic reactions for the first time.
- The most common allergy irritants are:
  - pollens
  - animal dander (shed by dogs, cats, horses, rabbits)
  - house dust
  - feathers in pillows, comforters, down-filled cushions
  - foods: nuts, shellfish
  - insect bites
  - industrial chemicals

Helpful hints
→ Saline (saltwater) nose sprays are the only ones safe to use during pregnancy.

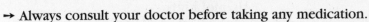

→ Always consult your doctor before taking any medication.
→ Don't take any cold or allergy medicine containing antihistamines (like Dristan, Contac, Allerest).
→ Consult your doctor early in your pregnancy if you have severe allergies. Asthmatic attacks or an anaphylactic reaction can deprive your baby of oxygen.
→ Stay indoors when pollen counts are high.
→ Air-condition your house and car to help filter the air.
→ Keep your house as dust-free as possible.
→ Buy electric air filters for the rooms you're in most.
→ Use hypoallergenic bed pillows and bedding.
→ Don't smoke or spend time in a smoke-filled room.

BABY HICCUPING

Causes and symptoms
● It is quite common for babies to get hiccups in the last half of your pregnancy.
● It does not cause discomfort for your baby—even if the hiccups last fifteen minutes or more.

Helpful hints
Just relax and enjoy your baby's movements!

BABY KICKING

Signs and symptoms
● By the fifth month of your pregnancy you will feel your baby kicking. The amount of movement experienced varies from pregnancy to pregnancy.
● The fetus is usually most active when you are at rest—either at night or before rising in the morning.
● Some babies have a regular pattern of kicking, others are inconsistent.

Helpful hints
→ If the kicking is particularly uncomfortable, try shifting your position.
→ Report to your doctor immediately if there's a big drop in movement during any twenty-four-hour period after the thirtieth week.

BACKACHE

Signs and symptoms
- Backache, especially later in pregnancy, is the result of the increased weight you're carrying.
- Lower backache can result from walking and sitting improperly.

Helpful hints
→ Don't stand in one position for too long. If you cannot move around, then put one foot forward with all your weight on it and then switch to the other leg.
→ Lean forward when standing at the kitchen counter, ironing board, etc. Bend your knees slightly and support your weight on your hands or elbows.
→ Pelvic rock relieves backache. (Kneel on all fours with your elbows straight, legs slightly apart. Inhale as you curl your back up and tuck your head under, exhale as you relax your back.) Do the exercise twenty times before lying down to rest or sleep.
→ While you're asleep put a small pillow under your side at waist level. This keeps your shoulders and hips in proper alignment.
→ Putting a footstool under your feet while you're sitting can relieve backache. Your knees should be at a slightly higher level than your hips.
→ To ease lower backache, tuck in your buttocks and abdomen every time you rise from sitting. Good posture when you walk is also insurance against lower backache.

BLEEDING AND SPOTTING

Causes and symptoms
- Pink-stained or red-streaked mucus that occurs right after inter-course or a vaginal examination is normal.
- Brownish tinged mucus or spotting occurring forty-eight hours after intercourse or vaginal examination is normal.

Helpful hints
Call your doctor if you have doubts or there is more bleeding than that described above.

BODY CHANGES

Permanent changes
- Area around nipple may darken and get broader.
- Shoe size increases by half a size.
- Dark line from belly button down abdomen.
- Darkening of the genitalia.
- Stretch marks may appear on abdomen, thighs, breasts.

Temporary changes
- Blood volume increases by 25 percent, causing heart to work harder.
- All ligaments in body stretch.
- Breasts get larger; veins more prominent.
- Lungs work more efficiently.
- Digestive system uses food more efficiently.

BREASTS

Signs and symptoms
- Your breasts will swell during pregnancy—sometimes as much as three cup sizes. This is because the milk glands are beginning to develop.

- The veins become more prominent because of the increased blood supply to the breasts.
- The *areola* (the area around the nipples) may darken and spread due to hormonal changes.
- Nipple secretion is common later in pregnancy.
  - This sticky, yellowish, watery fluid is *colostrum,* which will be the baby's first food. It comes in before your milk supply.
  - As the due date nears the secretion becomes whitish and resembles milk.
  - Colostrum may be gently expressed from the nipples if you wish.

Helpful hints
- Wear a support bra all through your pregnancy. For women whose breasts get very large it is a good idea to wear a bra even at night. This will help prevent sagging.
- Lumpy breasts are quite common in pregnancy.
- If a breast lump feels suspicious in any way—if it is hard or fixed or causes dimpling of the overlying skin—talk to your doctor.
- In some cases it may be wise to screen for breast cancer.
  - This can be done in pregnancy with diaphanography, which causes no harm to the fetus.
  - This method illuminates the breast with light.
  - A biopsy of the breast during pregnancy can be necessary if there is a suspicious lump. This is not dangerous for the fetus.

CONSTIPATION

Signs and symptoms
- Constipation, caused by the pressure of the uterus on the bowels, is a common complaint of pregnancy.
- The increased level of progesterone in your system relaxes the muscles, which makes the bowels less efficient.
- The proper definition of constipation is the passing of hard stool, not having infrequent bowel movements. Every second or third day may be sufficient for many women.
- As long as the stools aren't loose, watery, or bloody, there is no need to be worried.

Helpful hints

→ Eat plenty of fresh fruit. Apples have the greatest laxative action, along with dried fruits like prunes, figs, dates, and raisins.

→ Green vegetables add roughage to your diet. Raw or lightly cooked vegetables with skins left on are best.

→ Drink at least six to eight glasses of fluids a day.

→ Fiber from whole-grain breads and cereals will help stimulate your intestines.

→ Exercise, even if it's only walking, helps constipation.

→ Licorice candy can sometimes give relief.

→ Natural-fiber laxatives have none of the drawbacks of chemical laxatives and can be used as often as you want. Metamucil is one brand name.

→ Regularity is important. Establishing a set time to move your bowels can alleviate constipation.

→ Some people find it easier to move their bowels if their feet are elevated while sitting on the toilet (this releases the anus).

DAIRY INTOLERANCE

Signs and symptoms

● Milk is recommended for pregnant women because of the calcium it contains.

● If you cannot tolerate milk, or if you just dislike the taste, there are plenty of ways to get the calcium you need (see "If You Can't Tolerate Milk" on page 42).

Helpful hints

→ There is very little lactose in natural cheeses, especially fermented cheeses. Try eating those.

→ Cultured milk products like yogurt and buttermilk (brands without added milk solids) have reduced amounts of lactose.

→ Many people with lactose intolerance (difficulty in digesting the milk sugar lactose) are able to tolerate other dairy products such as Lactaid milk, which has 70 percent of the lactose converted to a more easily digestible form.

DIZZINESS, FAINTNESS

Signs and symptoms
- Dizziness is most common in the second trimester, when your enlarged uterus presses on major blood vessels, causing a blood pressure drop.
- Low blood sugar from going too long without food can also be a cause of dizziness.

Helpful hints
→ Move slowly and always get up gradually to avoid creating blood pressure changes.

→ Eat more frequent, smaller meals.

→ Carry snacks such as pieces of fruit or raisins to raise your blood sugar.

→ If you are in a crowded or warm environment get out into the fresh air or open a window.

→ Make sure you are not wearing restrictive clothing. Wear clothes that are loose around the neck and waist.

→ If you feel light-headed or think you are going to faint, lie down with your feet elevated, or sit with your head between your knees until the dizziness passes.

→ Fainting is rare, and even if it happens it will not harm your baby.

→ Report any dizziness to a doctor and let him decide whether it is a sign of a problem.

FATIGUE

Signs and symptoms
- Fatigue is most pronounced in early pregnancy, when your body may need several hours more sleep a day.
- Your body is making the necessary adjustments to pregnancy. Once it has adjusted and the placenta is complete (around the fourth month) you should have more energy.

- Fatigue is increased in the first trimester by a deficiency in iron or protein. Make sure that you are filling all your nutritional requirements.
- Common signs of fatigue are: impatience, irritability, inability to concentrate, and loss of interest in sex.

Helpful hints

→ Don't fight the fatigue. Think of it as your baby asserting his needs!
→ Go to bed earlier or take naps. Even five or ten minutes with your feet up and your eyes closed can be refreshing.
→ Let other people relieve you of some of your chores.
→ Listen to what your body is telling you. Pace yourself. Overexertion can harm your baby.
→ If you continue to be fatigued even after careful resting, tell your doctor. It may be a sign of anemia.

FOOD: AVERSIONS AND CRAVINGS

Causes and symptoms

- Tastes for certain foods do change during pregnancy.
- It was once believed that food cravings steered us toward foods the body needed. The fact is, these signals are unreliable.
- Most cravings and aversions disappear by the fourth month.

Helpful hints

→ You can't ignore a food aversion, but if you can't face foods from important food groups you should try to compensate for the nutrients they supply.
→ If you crave something that you know is not good for you, try to find a satisfactory replacement
→ Pickles, potato chips, and other salty foods that are often the objects of pregnancy cravings will make you retain water.

GAS PAINS

Causes and symptoms
- Gas is a common complaint of pregnancy.
- The stomach and intestines distend and you get a bloated feeling.

Helpful hints
→ Milk of magnesia after each meal increases intestinal activity, which may reduce gas.
→ Avoid gas-producing foods like beans, parsnips, corn, onions, cabbage, fried foods, sweet desserts, and candy.
→ Pureed vegetables may give additional relief.
→ Regular bowel movements reduce gas.

GROIN PAINS

Signs and symptoms
- Groin pains are mild, achy sensations in one or both sides of your abdomen.
- They are probably due to stretching of the ligaments that support the uterus.

Helpful hints
Gentle exercise for stretching may help.

HAIR AND NAILS

Signs and symptoms
- Changes caused by pregnancy hormones will lead to increased growth of nails and hair.

- Hair can also become more or less oily, just like your skin.
- You may find your hair has more or less body while you are pregnant.

Helpful hints
→ Do not use hair dye when you're pregnant. Permanent hair dyes can enter the bloodstream: the health implications are unclear.
→ If your hair is oily, try changing your shampoo or wash your hair more frequently, scrubbing the scalp vigorously.
→ For dry hair, wash less frequently and use moisturizing conditioner.

HEADACHES

Signs and symptoms
- Headaches are common during pregnancy.
- They're a result of the changes your body is going through. Pregnancy hormones may cause congestion of the mucous membranes, making sinus headaches common.
- There are many nondrug remedies for headaches.

Helpful hints
→ *DO NOT TAKE ASPIRIN DURING PREGNANCY.* It may be harmful to your baby and cause complications during labor.
    🡄 Aspirin substitutes such as Tylenol and Anacin have only been used since the 1970s; long-term effects on the fetus are not yet known.
    🡄 Many over-the-counter medications contain aspirin and acetaminophen. Read all labels carefully.
    🡄 Ibuprofen (trade names Advil and Nuprin) can cause problems in the unborn baby and complications during labor.
    🡄 No medication should be taken without your physician's approval.
    🡄 See page 12 for more aspirin information.
→ Get plenty of rest. Lack of sleep can cause headaches.
→ Crowded and overheated rooms should be avoided. Get outside for some fresh air.
→ Eat regularly. Low blood sugar levels can cause headaches.

→ Tension is the most common cause of headaches.
  ⚘ Lying down in a quiet room will help.
  ⚘ Meditation and yoga are particularly effective in relieving tension.
→ Sinus headaches can be relieved by applying hot and cold compresses to the aching area. Experiment with what works best for you.
→ If the headache is persistent, severe, or is accompanied by visual problems, inform your practitioner.

HEARTBURN, INDIGESTION

Signs and symptoms
● Heartburn is a burning sensation in the chest, but it has nothing to do with the heart.
● Heartburn is caused when digestive fluid backs up from the stomach and irritates the lining of the esophagus.
● Indigestion in pregnancy is caused by increased amounts of progesterone and estrogen, which relax smooth muscle tissue everywhere in your body. They also relax the sphincter separating the esophagus from the stomach. The positive result is that food moves more slowly through your system. This allows food nutrients to be absorbed more efficiently.

Helpful hints
→ Avoid greasy or spicy foods.
→ Avoid large meals, especially right before going to bed.
→ Avoid alcohol.
→ Sleep propped up with your head elevated. That way stomach acid can't flow back up into your esophagus at night.
→ Sip milk, which coats and soothes the stomach.
→ Don't take bicarbonate of soda (baking soda), which has a high salt content and causes swelling.
→ Take liquid antacid or suck on antacid tablets.
→ Milk of magnesia is soothing after each meal and whenever heartburn occurs.

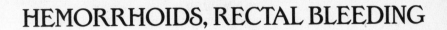

HEMORRHOIDS, RECTAL BLEEDING

Causes and symptoms

- Hemorrhoids are the result of the increased pressure on the veins in your anus.
- Hemorrhoids can be itchy, painful, and can cause bleeding.
- Rectal bleeding is often the result of cracks in the anus caused by constipation.

Helpful hints

→ Always consult a physician for proper diagnosis. Rectal bleeding is sometimes a sign of a more serious condition.

→ Don't allow yourself to get constipated, because straining and pushing worsens hemorrhoids. Use suppositories if necessary.

→ Do the Kegel exercise to stimulate circulation.

→ Twenty-five mg. of vitamin B_6 at each meal for several days may clear up the hemorrhoids entirely. Taking 10 mg. at every meal can help prevent a recurrence. As with any remedy, check first with your doctor.

→ Sit only on hard surfaces once you have hemorrhoids.

→ Yoga position: sit tailor-fashion on the floor, let your belly fall forward, taking weight off your pelvis and back. Once you get hemorrhoids it is helpful to sit this way whenever possible.

→ Cold compresses with witch hazel are comforting.

→ Put some petroleum jelly on a tissue, lie with your hips on a pillow, and gently push the hemorrhoid back into the rectum with the tissue. Stay with your hips elevated for about ten minutes, keeping the muscles surrounding the rectum tight.

ITCHY STOMACH

Causes and symptoms

- Pregnant stomachs are itchy. They can become more itchy as the pregnancy progresses.
- Your skin is stretching and the result is dryness and itching.

Helpful hints
→ Try to avoid scratching, which may only make you feel itchier.

→ Keeping the stomach well moisturized may help, but it probably won't eliminate the itchiness entirely.

MUSCLE CRAMPS

Causes and symptoms

• Muscle cramps are due to the slowing of your blood circulation.

• Another cause of cramping can be the sudden contraction of one of the two round ligaments that moor the uterus in front.

• Cold weather also seems to set off cramps in some women.

• Shooting pains down your legs can be due to pressure of the baby's head on certain nerves. This can be helped by changing your position.

Helpful hints

→ A heating pad, hot-water bottle, and massage all give relief.

→ Elevating the legs can prevent cramps.

→ Increase your intake of calcium and potassium.

    ✭ Put dried milk powder or bonemeal in a glass of milk before bed.

    ✭ Have a glass of milk before bed with 10 to 25 mg. of vitamin B_6 and two to three tablets of combined calcium and magnesium.

    ✭ To increase your potassium intake eat half a grapefruit or orange or banana before meals or as a snack.

→ To relieve leg cramps: while sitting or lying, force your toes back toward your face and push down on the knee at the same time to straighten your leg.

NAUSEA

Causes and symptoms

- Nausea is the most common complaint of the first three months of pregnancy.
- The higher level of estrogen in your system influences even the stomach cells and causes irritation as acids accumulate.
- Another reason for nausea is the rapid expansion of the uterus.
- Early morning is worst because stomach acids have accumulated and blood sugar is low after hours without food.

Helpful hints

→ To prevent low blood sugar eat some protein and a little natural starch or natural sugar (milk or cheese with fruit or juice) immediately before going to bed.

→ Keep crackers, popcorn, or dry toast by your bedside. Nibble some before you even raise your head in the morning. Remain lying down for twenty minutes before you get up.

→ At breakfast, go easy on food containing fats. Eat fruit or fruit juice (which are acidic) at the *end* of the meal.

→ Vitamin B$_6$ (pyridoxine) may have antinauseant properties. Ask your doctor about taking 50 mg. of B$_6$ daily.

→ Eating a diet high in protein and carbohydrates can help fight nausea.

→ Never let your stomach get empty. It's harder to eat once you're nauseated.

    ❧ Have five or six smaller meals instead of three large ones.

    ❧ Nibble on nutritious foods between meals.

    ❧ Get in the habit of keeping snacks nearby so you can keep something in your stomach all the time.

→ Avoid greasy or spicy foods.

→ Absolutely avoid coffee or sweets.

→ Experiment with drinking very hot or very cold liquids. The extreme temperatures may make you feel better.

→ Get extra sleep and give yourself relaxation time. Emotional and physical fatigue both increase morning sickness.

→ Drink plenty of fluids, particularly if you're losing them through vomiting. (Ginger ale and *nondiet* colas are valuable; they're rich in carbohydrates and the carbonation can often help, too).

→ Medication: if you absolutely cannot keep food down, your doctor may prescribe medication. Many antinausea drugs have been found dangerous in the past. Any risk has to be weighed against the benefit of providing essential nutrients for your baby that are lost if you can't keep anything down.

NOSEBLEEDS

Causes and symptoms

- Nosebleeds occur in pregnancy as a result of the increased blood volume.
- You may also have nasal congestion, which may be caused by the increased hormone levels in your body.
- Stuffiness will usually last until after you deliver. You may develop a postnasal drip, which can occasionally lead to night-time coughing.

Helpful hints

→ Vaseline will stop the bleeding if you put a little in each nostril.
→ Eat citrus fruits and other sources of vitamin C because a vitamin C deficiency may be the cause of the nosebleeds.
→ Make a 25 percent solution of menthol in white oil. Lubricate each nostril with a few drops, using an eye dropper. Tip your head back so the menthol runs into your throat, then spit it out. An application in the morning and another in the evening should stop nosebleeds.
→ Increase your fluid intake to compensate for any loss due to sneezing or a runny nose.
→ *DO NOT USE NOSE DROPS.* The side effects can be harmful to the baby. Besides, the excessiveness of nose drops can make the condition worse.

OVERHEATING

Causes and symptoms

- Your metabolic rate increases 20 percent during pregnancy, and as a result you're likely to feel warmer, even in the winter, when everyone else is cold!

- You may perspire more as your body attempts to cool you off and rid your body of waste products.

Helpful hints
→ Wear layers so you can peel them off when you start to feel hot.
→ Bathe more often and choose an effective antiperspirant.
→ Drink enough to replace the fluids you lose through your perspiration.

PINS AND NEEDLES

Causes and symptoms
- You may experience pins and needles in your hands and feet. This may give you the impression that your circulation is being cut off, but it isn't.
- No one really knows what causes this condition or how to prevent it. However, it is not an indication of anything serious.

Helpful hints
→ Changing your position may help.
→ If you experience swelling of your hands you may be developing "carpal tunnel syndrome."
  - This condition places pressure on a nerve in the wrist, causing a burning sensation that may radiate up the arm.
  - The symptoms may increase at night because fluids have accumulated in your hands all day, increasing swelling.
  - Ask your doctor whether you could be developing this condition and request information about possible treatments.

SALIVA, EXCESS

Cause and symptoms
- Excessive salivation can accompany nausea. It usually occurs in the first trimester, but happens rarely.

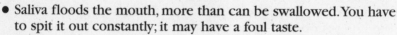

- Saliva floods the mouth, more than can be swallowed. You have to spit it out constantly; it may have a foul taste.
- It begins two to three weeks after your first missed period and can persist throughout the pregnancy.

Helpful hints
→ Foods containing starch aggravate this condition. As a first step eliminate all of the many vegetable foods containing starch.
→ Mild sedatives may help.
→ Strong mouthwashes or sucking peppermint candies may give relief.

SHORTNESS OF BREATH

Causes and symptoms
- Shortness of breath sometimes goes along with dizziness and feeling faint.
- Your respiration is deeper now, which allows you to take in more air and use it more efficiently. Your lungs have more space because the rib cage increases in size.
- The increase in the size of your rib cage is permanent. You may need a larger bra or blouse size even after you lose every pound you gained during pregnancy.

Helpful hints
→ Take three or four deep breaths before getting up from a sitting or lying position.
→ Consciousness of the need to breathe is a common experience in pregnancy. Move around or take a walk to alleviate the feeling.
→ Shortness of breath can be worse in the last weeks of pregnancy. The expanding uterus is largest then and presses on the diaphragm. If it gets too uncomfortable you can sleep propped with pillows in a semi-sitting position.

SKIN PROBLEMS

Your skin is affected by pregnancy. It's important to avoid picking or fussing with any of these skin conditions. Most skin problems will disappear after the pregnancy (with the exception of stretch marks and darkening of the genitalia, which occur in some women).

CONDITION	CAUSE	CURE
Pimples	If your skin breaks out before your period you will probably get pimples now because similar hormones are active in your system.	Keep your skin clean. *Avoid makeup.* When you do use foundation use a water-based product. Drink plenty of water. If your doctor approves, take vitamin B_6 supplement (25–50 mg.).
Bumps on your skin	Caused by normal hormonal changes in your blood.	Bumps will disappear after the baby is born.
Tiny red marks	Caused by distended blood vessels that rise to the surface of the skin.	They will disappear after the baby is born.
Brown spots on your face, neck, and abdomen	Often called the "mask of pregnancy," these spots may indicate a folic acid deficiency.	They will usually clear in the month following delivery. Taking 5 mg. of folic acid per meal will restore normal skin within two to three weeks, but check with your doctor first.
Dark nipples	In many women the areola (area around the nipple) darkens around the third month due to hormonal changes.	This darkening is permanent and will not go away after pregnancy.
Stretch marks	The result of scar tissue forming wherever normal elasticity is lacking, affecting 90 percent of pregnant women. Some authorities say you can prevent them.	Get adequate protein in your diet and take vitamin C and E supplements with your doctor's approval. Keep skin supple: Use oil or cream of cocoa butter daily.

SLEEP PROBLEMS

Causes and symptoms

- Sleep is affected in some way for all pregnant women.
- As your stomach grows bigger you may find it increasingly difficult to get comfortable. You might have to adjust your normal sleeping position.

Helpful hints

→ Do not sleep on your back; this puts all your weight on your internal organs and can also aggravate hemorrhoids.
  - Sleep on your side with one leg crossed over and a pillow between your legs or under the "crossover" leg to improve circulation.
→ Your bed should be large; in late pregnancy even a double bed may not be big enough for comfort.
  - Invest in a queen- or king-size bed if at all possible; later on a larger bed will permit you to breast-feed comfortably in bed.
→ Try a foam mattress pad if you can't get comfortable in the later stages of pregnancy.
  - Your body may need a surface that has more give.
  - A softer surface may help you sleep better.

STUFFY NOSE

Causes and symptoms

- Nasal stuffiness is a normal side effect of pregnancy. If you already have allergies they can be aggravated now.
- You may also find that a stuffy nose, watery eyes, or other allergic reactions happen to you for the first time when you're pregnant.

Helpful hints

→ Breathe steam:
  - Take a steam bath or steam shower.
  - Stand in a very hot shower, breathing deeply.
  - Put a few drops of eucalyptus oil into a pot of very hot water. Lean over the pot with a towel draped over your head and breathe deeply, allowing the steam to help clear the blocked sinuses.

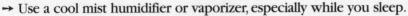

- → Use a cool mist humidifier or vaporizer, especially while you sleep.
- → Cover your nose with a hot washcloth to soothe sinuses.
- → Massage your sinuses using finger pressure firmly around your eyes.
- → Drink hot liquids.
- → Do not take any kind of antihistamine or cold remedy (Dristan, Contac, Allerest, Coricidin). They have caused birth defects in test animals.
- → Use only *saline* (saltwater) nasal sprays.

SWEATING

Causes and symptoms
- ● Sweating may increase when you're pregnant as your thyroid gland becomes more active.
- ● You also manufacture more heat when you're pregnant. Your body has to sweat more to maintain your body temperature.
- ● Sweat also serves to dispose of additional waste material in your system.

Helpful hints
- → If you develop any irritation, powder yourself with cornstarch or a medicated powder.
- → Sweating may be excessive at night; if so, put a towel on your pillow.

SWELLING (EDEMA)

Causes and symptoms
- ● Swelling (edema) is a *normal* condition affecting around 40 percent of pregnant women.
- ● It is particularly common late in the day, in warm weather, or after you have been sitting or standing a lot.

- Swelling is a result of the rise of hormones that normally cause fluid retention (as they do before your period).
- Studies have shown that women with edema have slightly larger babies—and fewer premature babies—than those without edema.

Helpful hints

→ Anything more than mild edema—or if edema persists for more than a day—should be reported immediately to your doctor.
  - Severe edema can be a sign that you have kidney problems or other complications.
→ Diuretics (water pills) are harmful during pregnancy. They cause a potassium deficiency, which in turn causes fatigue, mental depression, and insomnia, and can be harmful to the kidneys.
→ Vitamin C increases urine production and can be effective in removing excess fluids. Ask your doctor.
→ Vitamin B_6 is an effective diuretic, particularly when used with vitamin C. Vitamin B_6 can sometimes upset the stomach, so take it with food or milk if your doctor okays it.
→ A high-protein diet can help drive the extra fluid out of your system.
→ Mild and frequent exercise such as swimming and walking helps edema.
→ Avoid high-salt foods: you'll get a better result by increasing your protein intake and continuing to salt your food to taste.
→ Avoid tight clothes that are constricting at the waist or wrists.
→ Remove rings if your fingers get puffy.
  - If your hands have already swollen it may be difficult to get the rings off.
  - Soak your hand in cold water, then hold the finger pointing upward. Soap your finger and the ring before attempting to remove the ring.
→ Avoid standing in one position for a long time: move around to help your circulation.
→ Tired feet and swollen ankles can be helped in several ways.
  - Immerse your feet in cold water.
  - Rolling or rotating your ankles reduces swelling.
  - Put support panty-hose on before you get up in the morning, before the swelling starts.
→ Swelling of the vaginal area can be uncomfortable. A cold compress held against the swollen area will help.
→ Drink at least eight to ten eight-ounce glasses of liquids daily.

TEETH AND GUMS

Causes and symptoms

- Teeth and gums can be affected by your pregnancy.
- Hormonal changes can exaggerate the response of periodontal tissue to plaque.
  - These changes can also decrease your body's immune response to bacteria.
  - Bacteria can enter your bloodstream and infections can cross the placenta.
  - Any infective source should be eliminated.
- There is a greater susceptibility to gum problems, especially in the upper jaw. Your susceptibility increases during pregnancy: it's greatest in the eighth month and then decreases.
- Bleeding gums may occur because the increased blood volume puts pressure on the capillaries.

Helpful hints

→ Diet helps prevent tooth and gum problems. Sufficient calcium and high-quality protein along with a good supply of vitamins C, B, and D should protect you.
→ Floss and brush regularly. To further reduce bacteria, brush your tongue when you brush your teeth.
→ See the dentist at least once during your pregnancy and have your teeth cleaned professionally.

URINATING FREQUENTLY

Causes and symptoms

- In the first months of pregnancy the hormonal changes in your body send you to the bathroom more often.
- Your kidneys are working more effectively, clearing the waste products from the body more rapidly.
- Another reason for the need to urinate frequently is that your bladder is pressed by the growing uterus.

- As your baby settles into the pelvic cavity (engagement), it will put additional pressure on your bladder.
  - In a first pregnancy this can happen two to four weeks before delivery.
  - In later pregnancies engagement may not occur until labor begins.

Helpful hints
→ Do not restrict fluid intake to lessen the problem of frequent urination. Your body needs additional fluids when it is working for two.
→ Increased urination at night is caused by water retained in your ankles during the day, which moves to your kidneys.
→ One way to cut down midnight trips to the bathroom is not to drink any liquids after 7:00 P.M.

URINARY TRACT INFECTION (UTI)

Causes and symptoms
- Urinary infections are more common during pregnancy, when your body is more susceptible to any kind of bacteria.
- Cystitis is the most common bladder infection. You have the urge to urinate every five minutes, only to pass a few drops, maybe with a burning sensation.
- Pyelitis is a kidney infection.
  - The normal path of urine elimination is blocked and waste material backs up into your body.
  - Symptoms are similar to those of cystitis but may be accompanied by a high temperature, chills, and blood in the urine.

Helpful hints
→ At the first sign of a UTI, notify your doctor. S/he will prescribe one of the antibiotics approved for use during pregnancy.
→ Drink plenty of water.
→ Wear cotton underwear and avoid tight under or outer pants.

→ Keep the vaginal area clean.
  - Wash with unperfumed soaps.
  - Always wipe from front to back after using the toilet.

VAGINAL DISCHARGE

Causes and symptoms

- Pregnancy increases the activity of the mucus-secreting glands of the cervix so there's an increase in vaginal discharge.
- The discharge may increase until the baby is due, becoming quite heavy in some women.
- There may also be an increase in vaginal odor.

Helpful hints

→ Wear a light sanitary pad.
→ Keep the genital area clean and dry but don't overdo cleaning with soap, which could be irritating.
→ Douching will not lessen the discharge and it gives only temporary relief for odor. It is the secretions themselves that have a strong odor.
  - Some doctors advise against douching during pregnancy, so check with your doctor.
  - Never douche if you have had vaginal bleeding at any time during your pregnancy.
  - Do not douche during the last month of pregnancy.
  - Insert the nozzle no more than two inches inside the lips of your vagina.
  - Never hold the labia (the lips of the vagina) together; the water has to flow out freely.

VARICOSE VEINS

Causes and symptoms

- Increased blood volume and blood flow during pregnancy place pressure on the pelvic and leg veins, causing the veins to bulge.
- Later in pregnancy the baby's head also presses down on the pelvic veins.
- Varicose veins are hereditary.
- Varicose veins do get worse with subsequent pregnancies, so do everything you can to keep your condition under control.

Helpful hints

→ Elevate your legs when you're lying down or resting, preferably raising them above the level of your heart.

→ Wear support panty-hose or elastic support stockings. Put them on before you get out of bed in the morning; take them off before you go to sleep.

→ Exercise regularly. A long, brisk walk every day can help.

→ Vitamins C and E can help prevent or control varicose veins. However, consult your doctor before attempting any vitamin therapy on your own.

→ Don't gain too much weight; excessive weight gain causes the veins to dilate.

→ Don't stand or sit still for long periods of time; try to keep moving around.

→ The lips of your vagina can develop varicose veins too.

  - Sleep with your bottom raised up on a pillow.
  - Wear a sanitary pad pressed firmly against the swollen part of your vulva.
  - Talk to your obstetrician about a "maternity garment" that compresses the vulva by putting pressure on the perineal area. This custom-made vascular support is made by companies like the Jobst Institute (1-800-537-1063) and requires a doctor's prescription.

VOMITING

Causes and symptoms

- Vomiting, like nausea, diminishes as your pregnancy continues.
- You may throw up in the morning, in the evening, or at irregular times.
- Do not be concerned by blood flecks or streaks if you have been vomiting fairly often.
  - Repeated vomiting may rupture a tiny blood vessel in the throat or esophagus.
  - This soon clots or heals by itself.

Helpful hints

- Vitamin B_6 can help control vomiting. Once vomiting has begun, 250 mg. a day or more is necessary, or your doctor could give you a 300mg. or larger injection of vitamin B_6 if the vomiting is severe. Ask his or her opinion.
- Dehydration and loss of calories is a danger with repeated vomiting.
- Hyperemesis gravidarum is a rare complication of pregnancy.
  - It is severe and unremitting vomiting that can be controlled only with antiemetic drugs and hospitalization.
  - Most frequent in women with abnormally high hormone levels, as happens in cases of multiple births or placental abnormalities.
  - This illness is seen most frequently in pregnant women who are under emotional stress, which suggests that emotions may play a part in the disorder.

DANGER SIGNS DURING PREGNANCY

(Possible cause for symptoms in parentheses)

- PAIN OR BURNING ON URINATION (urinary tract infection; sexually transmitted disease)
- VAGINAL SPOTTING OR BLEEDING (premature labor; miscarriage; placenta previa or abruptio)
- LEAKING OR GUSHING FLUID FROM VAGINA, less significant near due date (rupture of membranes)
- BLISTER OR SORE IN VAGINAL AREA, itching or irritating discharge (vaginal infection; sexually transmitted disease)
- UTERINE CONTRACTIONS, more than four or five in an hour not near your due date (threatened miscarriage)
- SEVERE NAUSEA OR VOMITING, several times in an hour or over several days (hyperemesis gravidarum; infection)
- SEVERE ABDOMINAL PAIN (ectopic pregnancy; placenta abruptio; premature labor)
- CHILLS AND FEVER OVER 100°F. not accompanied by a common cold (infection)
- DIZZINESS OR LIGHT-HEADEDNESS (toxemia)
- SEVERE HEADACHE that doesn't let up, especially in the second half of pregnancy (toxemia)
- SWELLING OF FACE, EYES, FINGERS, OR TOES, especially if the puffiness is sudden (toxemia)
- SUDDEN WEIGHT GAIN (toxemia)
- VISUAL PROBLEMS: dimness, blurring, spots, flashes, blind spots (toxemia)
- NOTICEABLY REDUCED FETAL MOVEMENT (fetal distress)
- ABSENCE OF FETAL MOVEMENT FOR 24 HOURS from 30th week of pregnancy and beyond (fetal death)
- A HOT, REDDENED PAINFUL AREA BEHIND YOUR KNEE or on your calf (phlebitis or blood clot)

5.
Prenatal Diagnosis

Tests—What to Have and When to Have Them

AMNIOCENTESIS

Reasons for amniocentesis
- To discover whether the fetus has a chromosomal abnormality.
- If you have a previous child with a metabolic defect, "amnio" can detect defects in other unborn children.
- Late in pregnancy "amnio" can confirm if the baby is mature enough to be delivered if there are medical reasons to induce labor.

How is it done?
- A needle is inserted through your stomach and a small amount of amniotic fluid is withdrawn.
- The procedure is usually painless. A local anesthetic can be used if you have discomfort.

When is it done?
- Normally, 14 to 16 weeks after your last menstrual period.
- Results take 2 to 4 weeks.

Risk?
- There is a very small risk to the fetus and/or you, in the unlikely event there are complications from the biopsy needle.
- Women under thirty-five are usually not given amniocentesis (however, 85 percent of Down's babies are born to women under thirty-five).

CHORIONIC VILLUS SAMPLING (CVS)

What does CVS reveal?
- Genetic defects
- Chromosomal abnormalities
- Metabolic conditions
- Blood-borne problems and defects

How is it done?
- A catheter is guided by ultrasound through your cervix and into your uterus.
- A sample of chorionic villi tissue is withdrawn. CVS is not part of the fetus but contains fetal tissue.

When is it done?
- Usually in the ninth or tenth week.
- Results are available in a day or two.

Risks?
- As with amniocentesis, there is a small but significant risk to the fetus because a biopsy needle is inserted into the womb.
- There is a slightly higher risk of miscarriage with CVS than with amniocentesis.

Drawbacks
- CVS is slightly less accurate than "amnio" for detecting chromosomal abnormalities like Down's syndrome.
- CVS cannot detect neural tube defects (like spina bifida). However, you can compensate for this with a blood serum test in week sixteen.
- There is also a small risk of false positive results. The test can *mistakenly* indicate there is something wrong with the baby. If you have the misfortune of getting a positive CVS, talk to your doctor about the need to reconfirm the accuracy of the test result.

ULTRASOUND

What does ultrasound reveal?
- Helps determine your due date by showing the baby's size.
- Shows if there is more than one baby.
- Identifies fetal disorders like fluid on the brain.
- Discovers tumors in the uterus and ectopic pregnancies.
- Monitors your baby's growth, movements, breathing, and heart rate.
- Can show fetal death.

How is it done?
- An ultrasound is a painless and risk-free procedure.
- High-frequency sound waves are beamed toward the baby, projecting an image on a monitor screen.
- Pictures are made of the image as a permanent record.

When is it done?
At various times during the pregnancy, depending on individual circumstances.

ALPHA FETOPROTEIN TESTING (AFP)

What does AFP reveal?
- Some birth defects
- An early warning of potentially dangerous conditions
- Neural tube defects such as spina bifida
- The presence of more than one child
- Low birth weight
- Fetal death

How and when is it done?
- A simple blood test at approximately sixteen weeks.
- A high level of AFP is a warning sign. The test can then be repeated to follow the baby's condition.
- If the blood levels remain high an ultrasound scan is done.

BLOOD AND CELL TESTS

What do they reveal?
- These tests are new and with research are being improved all the time.
- Can find many more flaws than previous tests, including the classic form of hemophilia.
- Testing is now fairly accurate for detecting muscular dystrophy.

Where are these tests done?
- The National Genetics Foundation (555 West 57th Street, New York, New York 10019) has a free service for analyzing your family health history.
- If necessary, they can refer you to one of the fifty-five genetic counseling centers across the country.
- Only a few laboratories offer these specialized tests—and they are expensive.

6.
What to Do During Pregnancy

*Exercise, Sex,
and Other Pastimes*

EXERCISE
DURING PREGNANCY

* Jogging one mile now can take as much effort as it did
  to go three miles before you were pregnant.
* Intense exercise is not advisable. If you're not usually an
  active person you won't change now ... but taking regular walks can be good for your circulation, digestion,
  and general health.

Guidelines for safe exercise during pregnancy
→ Moderate activity three times a week is a safe plan.
→ Exercise regularly, because exercising only sporadically
  can be a shock to your body.
→ Always stretch out your muscles and joints before
  starting.
→ Exercises should always be slow and rhythmic. Avoid
  jarring motions and excessive twisting of your joints.

→ Remember to breathe deeply throughout exercising: your body needs additional oxygen for your muscles to work properly and also for the baby.
→ Breathe through your nose as you relax and exhale through your mouth during the most difficult parts of any exercise.
→ During prolonged exercise the blood flow to your limbs deprives your baby of oxygen.
→ A full workout should last about thirty minutes, including ten minutes to warm up and another five to cool down.
→ Do not undertake any exercise without first checking with your healthcare provider.

KEGEL EXERCISES— WHAT'S SO IMPORTANT?

* If you do no other exercise during pregnancy, do this one!
* Kegels strengthen your pelvic floor muscles for labor and delivery and allow you to totally relax those muscles, which is very important during childbirth.
* Doing Kegels allows the vagina to regain its previous shape and muscle tone more quickly after birth.
* Once you recognize where these muscles are, you can exercise them regularly every day.

How to do the Kegel exercise
→ These are the same muscles used to stop the flow of urine. Get the feel of these muscles when you're urinating. Practice by stopping the flow of urine.
→ Think of an internal "elevator" to get a mental picture of the Kegel exercise.
→ Contract the muscles in small amounts, thinking of an elevator going up floors.
→ Contract the pelvic floor muscles as though you were going up in an elevator to the tenth floor.
→ Then release the muscular tension little by little, counting backward slowly down to one.

→ Releasing the contracted muscle is harder. Try to develop enough control so that you don't release the muscles completely until the "elevator" is fully back at the "first floor."

Where to do Kegels

→ They're easiest to do sitting down ... but once you get the hang of it you can do them standing or walking.
→ You can also do them lying down on your back with your knees bent and your feet on the floor a foot apart.
→ You can do the Kegels lying in bed or in a warm bath.
→ Lovemaking is a good time to practice:
   ⊷ When your partner's penis is inside you, suddenly tighten your pelvic floor muscles.
   ⊷ Hold that tension for as long as you can.
   ⊷ Your mate can feel how those muscles are developing as the pregnancy progresses.
→ Try to do about twenty-five Kegels at various times during the day.
→ This may seem a lot, but once you get into the habit, it will become something you do without any big mental effort.

Do Kegels immediately after birth

→ Continue to practice Kegels frequently after birth.
→ If you've had an episiotomy Kegels can help pull the stitches together and begin healing and strengthening the affected muscles.
→ In the first twenty-four hours after delivery you may not be able to feel yourself doing the exercise ... but it's doing you good.

WARNINGS ABOUT
EXERCISE DURING PREGNANCY

→ Never exercise to the point of fatigue: a pregnant woman's body can't bounce back easily from exercise.

→ Stop if you feel any pain during exercise. Use common sense and trust your body's signals.

→ How to tell if you're exerting yourself too much:

    ➤ While you're exercising you should be able to carry on a conversation comfortably.

    ➤ It's fine to perspire but if you're pouring with sweat you've gone too far.

    ➤ You've done too much if your pulse is still over 100 after a five-minute cooldown.

→ Avoid activities that raise your body temperature. Overheating can cause birth defects in the first trimester and can cause premature labor in the last trimester.

→ Treadmills and Stairmasters can elevate your body temperature and heart rate. Misuse of these machines can cause miscarriage or premature labor.

→ Don't exercise on an empty stomach: eat and drink lightly about half an hour beforehand.

→ Don't exercise flat on your back after the fourth month of pregnancy: this position compresses the artery that sends blood to your baby.

→ Avoid weight-bearing sports like backpacking.

→ Avoid any exercise that pulls on abdominal muscles. Nature is preparing your stomach muscles to separate to make room for the expanding uterus. Stomach exercises now can actually slow the recovery of abdominal tone after birth.

→ Slow down in the last trimester: don't push yourself beyond what feels good and easy.

BEST EXERCISES DURING PREGNANCY

Walking · It's best at a quick pace for about half an hour.

Swimming A great exercise because the water prevents you from straining or stressing joints and muscles.

Stationary bicycle As long as you pay attention to your posture and don't lean over the handlebars in a way that could give you a backache.

Pregnancy exercise classes Calisthenics designed specifically for pregnant women and conducted under supervision so you aren't straining your body without realizing it.

WORST EXERCISES DURING PREGNANCY

Scuba diving Circulation may be restricted by the equipment. Decompression sickness is dangerous for the fetus.

Horseback riding Unless you are an accomplished rider your center of gravity has changed and you're more likely to fall.

Downhill skiing Unless you are an extremely accomplished skier you may fall because your center of balance is off.

Jumping or diving into water Water could be forced into your vagina.

Waterskiing Again, unless you are an expert skier your balance is off, and a fall could force water into your vagina.

Skiing above 10,000 feet High altitude deprives you and the baby of all-important oxygen.

Bicycling in risky conditions There's a danger of falling in mountain biking on narrow paths or any biking on wet roads. A racing-type bicycle is a bad idea because you can get a backache from leaning over the handlebars.

Tennis in the last trimester As you get bigger your body cannot handle sudden moves; you also lose a sense of balance.

Calisthenics not specifically for pregnancy Avoid exercise videos or classes that are not geared to the needs of a pregnant body.

Jogging This is a hard exercise on your breasts, especially now that they are larger. It also jars your lower back and knees.

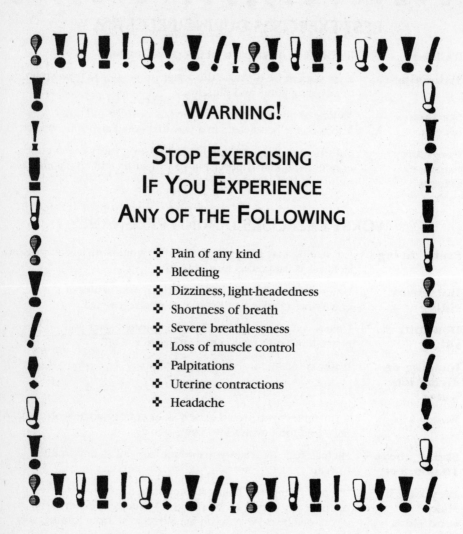

WARNING!

STOP EXERCISING
IF YOU EXPERIENCE
ANY OF THE FOLLOWING

- ✦ Pain of any kind
- ✦ Bleeding
- ✦ Dizziness, light-headedness
- ✦ Shortness of breath
- ✦ Severe breathlessness
- ✦ Loss of muscle control
- ✦ Palpitations
- ✦ Uterine contractions
- ✦ Headache

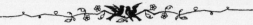

ANXIETIES ABOUT SEX

* Couples may feel anxious about the sexual aspect of pregnancy.
* If you can keep lines of communication open with each other, sex can be satisfying and fun.

Harming the baby
● Sex is not harmful for the baby. Nature has provided excellent cushioning (a woman can even fall down without harming the baby!).
● If either partner has any worries, talk to your doctor for reassurance.

Baby's reaction
● After lovemaking your baby may kick or squirm.
● This is a normal reaction to physical changes in your body.

Bringing on labor
● Some doctors routinely prohibit sex during the last six weeks of pregnancy. This may reinforce any fears you already have about sex.
● Labor will not start just because of uterine or cervical stimulation.
● It is true that if your body is ready for labor to begin, lovemaking *may* increase its progress.

YOUR FEELINGS
ABOUT YOUR BODY

Sex and your new body shape
● As your body grows you may feel undesirable. This can influence your feelings about sex.
● Most men are not negatively affected by a woman's pregnant body.
● Your partner may lose interest in sex for a variety of reasons during pregnancy—do not translate this as rejection.
● Talk about the changes your body is going through with your partner. It is really important to discuss your concerns with him.

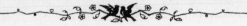

The last trimester
- By the last trimester you may be sick of being pregnant!
- You may just feel too huge and uncomfortable for lovemaking.
- Your fear of labor can upset you and make you withdraw sexually.

TALKING ABOUT SEX

Talking can make such a difference during pregnancy.
→ A lack of communication at this time can draw partners apart.
→ Sharing feelings helps you meet each others' needs.
→ Gentle reassurance is what both of you need from each other.
→ Communication can create a stronger, deeper, more trusting relationship.

Discuss your partner's feelings about your new body.
→ Changes in body shape and odor may turn your partner off.
→ The man may simply withdraw if you can't discuss it objectively and undefensively.
→ Sometimes expressing the negatives can diminish the feelings.

Discuss your feelings about your own body.
→ You may not feel good about your body.
→ Talk this out with your partner.
→ By resolving some of these feelings you will keep them from dominating your sex life.

Recognize the "dependency period."
→ About ten weeks before and after birth is when a pregnant woman needs the most support.
→ Sex can be helpful before childbirth because it alleviates tension as your due date nears.
→ Sex is also a way of "talking" to each other without words.

Sex can express unacknowledged feelings.
→ Refusing sex can be a way of expressing unmet needs or fears.
→ Having intercourse when you don't want to can produce morning sickness or other symptoms.
→ If you can't get satisfaction talking to your mate, consider professional counseling.

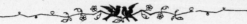

YOUR PARTNER'S FEELINGS ABOUT SEX

Your partner's reactions to your changing body, your increased (or decreased) eroticism, and the idea of parenthood all affect him sexually.

He may be overwhelmed.
- The changes in your body may be frightening to him.
- It's difficult for him to imagine all the changes you're going through and he may feel left out.

He may become temporarily impotent.
- Any of the above issues can leave a man unable to get an erection.
- Reassure your partner that this is not abnormal and will pass.
- Give him time to get used to everything that's going on.
- Think about ways to bolster his ego and self-esteem in nonsexual areas, which can give a boost to his sex drive.

He may feel inadequate sexually.
- If you are now more orgasmic he may worry that he cannot meet your increased sexual needs.
- If you are naturally more lubricated now, a man may feel his penis isn't "big enough."

He may feel guilty about sex gratification.
- There may be times when you're not interested in being sexually aroused now but want to give pleasure and sexual release to your partner.
- The man may feel you're having sex out of a sense of "duty."
- Encourage him to talk to you about his feelings.

WHY A MAN MIGHT HAVE LESS SEXUAL DESIRE

For different reasons, pregnancy can sometimes affect both partners' desire for sex.

Fear of hurting the fetus
→ It is not possible to hurt the baby during sex.
→ Men who still avoid sex despite this knowledge should talk to an obstetrician for reassurance that sex is safe.
→ However, a man's weight should never rest entirely on the woman without support of his arms.
→ For a few men, even knowing there's no danger does not put their minds at ease.

Guilt about "imposing" on the woman
→ A pregnant woman can often feel fatigue or other discomforts of pregnancy.
→ A man may back off from sex because it doesn't seem "fair" that he feels fine and has a healthy sex drive when his wife doesn't.
→ Nine months is too long to go without sex! Look for ways to reassure your mate that you love him and care about his gratification regardless of your temporary "slumps."

WHY YOU MAY HAVE LESS SEX DRIVE

Physical discomforts
→ Nausea or vomiting don't make you feel very sexy!
→ You may feel so fatigued you just collapse in an exhausted heap at night.
→ Other changes in your body may make you feel really uncomfortable or just sexually turned off.

Fears and anxieties

→ The anxieties and pressures of being pregnant may make you lose interest in sex.

→ Communicate these problems to your mate as soon as you're aware of them—or he may take your disinterest in sex as a disinterest in *him* sexually.

→ Both parents-to-be are very sensitive right now, so you each have to be protective of the other's vulnerability.

The last trimester of pregnancy

→ As your due date approaches much of your thought and energy are directed to preparing for the baby's birth.

→ It's natural to lose interest in sex during the last trimester—but unless the idea of sex makes you literally shudder, try to overcome your disinterest!

WHY YOU MAY WANT MORE SEX

Some women become highly erotic during pregnancy. Don't feel self-conscious about these feelings—share them with your mate.

No birth control
You feel mentally and physically free from worry about getting pregnant!

Hormones
Hormonal changes during pregnancy are similar to those of sexual arousal.

Breasts
Your bosoms are bigger and more sensitive to arousal.

Arousal
Women get turned on more rapidly and intensely.

Readiness
There is increased vaginal lubrication.

Orgasm
Some women reach orgasm for the first time during pregnancy.

SEX WITHOUT INTERCOURSE

Massage
→ Massage is an excellent way to communicate and express loving feelings.
→ Use a pleasantly scented oil, warming it in your hands before beginning.
→ If you feel the need, buy an illustrated massage manual.

Masturbation
→ Masturbation is an excellent way to relieve sexual tension.
→ Overcome hang-ups either of you might have before starting.
→ If you haven't practiced much manual or oral stimulation before pregnancy, encourage your partner to show and/or tell you what s/he likes.
→ *Mutual masturbation* is great when you want to share a sexual experience without intercourse.
→ *Using a vibrator* can add a fun and exciting dimension to manual stimulation. (It's not harmful to the baby.)
→ *Warning:* if you have spotting or pain, abstain from orgasm, which can be even more intense with masturbation than during intercourse.

ORGASMS

Experiencing orgasms for the first time
→ Orgasms can be one of the pleasant "side effects" of pregnancy!
→ Some women have their first orgasm when they are pregnant.

Having multiple orgasms
→ Increased blood flow to the genital area means an increase in your sexuality.
→ You may discover you have more than one orgasm.

Feeling aroused after the first orgasm and wanting to continue lovemaking
→ Don't be worried about becoming a sex maniac!
→ After birth sexuality returns to what it was pre-pregnancy.

Being unable to have an orgasm
→ Anxiety about labor and becoming a mother may make it difficult to relax and reach a climax.
→ Create a nondemanding atmosphere by agreeing to have sex *without* orgasms—just for the pleasure of caressing and kissing.
→ Remove the pressure for orgasm and you will not only enjoy sex again, you will probably have an orgasm before you know it.
→ It is normal to find yourself less orgasmic in the last trimester, as your due date nears.

Your genitals remain engorged.
→ After orgasm later in pregnancy you may be in a state of continued sexual tension.
→ Orgasm occasionally fails to relieve this tension.
→ Some women keep trying to have orgasms but don't feel release regardless of how much they come—the more they're stimulated, the longer this physical tension remains.

Uterine spasms after orgasm
→ In the third trimester you may experience uterine spasms instead of the usual rhythmic contractions you are accustomed to with orgasm.
→ Near term some women may have regularly recurring contractions for as long as half an hour after orgasm.
→ Early labor contractions are similar in rhythm and intensity to the uterine contractions of an orgasm.

Effects of orgasm on the fetus
→ Orgasm does cause a slight change in the fetal heart rate, but this does no harm.

BEST POSITIONS
FOR PREGNANT SEX

The growing baby will make you change your positions.
→ As your belly gets bigger you have to discover new ways to be comfortable during intercourse.
→ You want to eliminate pressure on your belly, which then can be caressed as a new erogenous zone.

Man on top but lying partly sideways
→ This position will carry you through most of your pregnancy because most of the man's weight is off you.

Woman on top
→ This position is comfortable for many people, especially because the woman can control how deep the penetration is.

Side positions
→ Either front-to-back or front-to-front are excellent during pregnancy.
→ A side position with the man behind so you fit together like "spoons" is good toward the end of pregnancy, when the woman's belly is largest.

BLEEDING AFTER SEX
IN THE FIRST THREE MONTHS

* Bleeding may be caused by a deep thrust that brings your partner's penis up against the cervix (the mouth of the uterus).
* The cervix is softer than usual and there is so much extra blood in the vessels that pressure may cause a small amount of bleeding.

Do not worry!
Such bruises, which are like nosebleeds, heal quickly.

Avoidance

The bleeding can be eliminated by avoiding deep penetration. It may help to have the woman on top so she can control penetration.

Check with your doctor.

If bleeding accompanies intercourse it may not be serious but you should consult your doctor to rule out the possibility of miscarriage or other problems.

SEX IN THE LAST TRIMESTER

This can be an awkward time sexually because your belly is big and you may generally have less energy.

You may want to avoid maximum penetration positions.

→ They may be uncomfortable.

→ You may also worry about the penis pressing on your cervix.

Women feel the need for increased affection.

→ As your due date approaches you may feel nervous and in need of reassurance.

→ Hugging and kissing not specifically related to sexual intercourse can meet this need.

You may wish to avoid sexual intercourse.

→ Talk to your mate about your feelings but don't force yourself to have sex if you're really uncomfortable about it.

→ See the section on sex without intercourse, page 134.

WHEN THE DOCTOR FORBIDS SEX

Sex is an important outlet for many feelings, including anger, anxiety, and insecurity. You may be conscious of these emotions and their connection to sexuality. Abstaining from sex may put extra pressure on your relationship at a time when it needs to be strong.

Does your doctor say to abstain?

→ Some doctors still routinely recommend abstaining from sex for the last six weeks of pregnancy.

→ Many doctors do not give a medical reason for this rule.

→ There are many doctors who don't put restrictions on a couple's sex life; some couples make love right up to delivery time.

→ Discuss any such orders with your doctor, don't just follow instructions without a medical necessity.

→ Consult another doctor if you are not fully convinced of your doctor's reasons for abstaining from sex.

→ The "warnings" box below outlines accepted reasons for banning sex.

WARNINGS!

Blowing air into the vagina
This unusual sexual activity could detach the placenta from the uterine wall. NOTE: This does not rule out oral sex.

The man's entire weight should never be on the woman
He should support himself with his arms if he's on top. Lying sideways also solves this problem. Great pressure should never be put on the uterus.

Reasons for no sex (at any time during pregnancy)
✤ Vaginal or abdominal pain
✤ Uterine pressure
✤ Membranes have ruptured
✤ You have been warned or think miscarriage might occur

◆◆◆◆◆◆◆◆◆◆◆◆◆◆◆◆◆◆◆◆◆◆◆◆◆

SEX AFTER THE BABY

After birth your body undergoes many adjustments. Your hormones have to level off and your uterus and vagina have to return to their normal size. Your vaginal area is also recovering from the trauma of childbirth. There's also pressure of a new baby in the house. All this puts a strain on the sexual aspect of your life.

THE BABY'S INFLUENCE ON SEX

The child can be felt as an intruder.
→ Your child may cry for your attention during intimate moments with your partner.
→ Learn to be flexible: try not to let the baby's demands put an end to whatever you were doing.
→ Do not allow yourself to give your child control of your life.

A woman can get overly absorbed in her baby.
→ You can be so satisfied with your attachment to the baby that you feel little need for other emotional ties.
→ Your partner may feel neglected: it is vitally important to remember his emotional needs.
→ By the end of the day you may be exhausted. By the time you put the baby down for the night you may have little energy left for your partner.
→ Let your partner know you're just feeling exhausted so he doesn't feel personally rejected.

BREAST-FEEDING AND SEX

Increased sexual stimulation
→ Some women find that nursing puts them more in touch with their bodies, which can heighten their sexuality.
→ The hormone produced during nursing is a sexual stimulant.
→ The baby's suckling can often produce sexual stimulation up to and sometimes including orgasm.
→ Many women feel guilty about becoming aroused. Relax. Think of it as a bonus to motherhood!

◆◆◆◆◆◆◆◆◆◆◆◆◆◆◆◆◆◆◆◆◆◆◆◆◆

FEELING LESS SEXY

Lower estrogen levels

→ It's quite normal not to want sex or not to be turned on easily after childbirth.

→ Lower estrogen levels can mean a lowered interest in sex.

→ Knowing there's a physical reason can prevent your partner from feeling rejected.

PHYSICAL CHANGES AND SEX

Your body's adjustment

→ For several months after birth your vaginal walls are thin and lubrication is sparse.

→ Use unscented K-Y jelly, or a similar product, if you have this problem.

→ You may feel better after your first period.

The diaphragm

→ Your diaphragm has to be refitted after childbirth. You will probably need a larger size.

→ Insertion may be difficult and painful soon after childbirth.

Exhaustion

→ It takes your body a full six weeks to recover from childbirth.

→ You also have to adjust to the demands of your baby.

Hormones

→ Your body needs time to return to a hormonal balance.

→ A woman may need extra fondling, kissing, and other foreplay to become aroused.

Leaking milk

→ You may lose breast milk in uncontrollable spurts when you are sexually aroused and during orgasm.

→ Don't let the leaking be a turn off to either of you.

→ There isn't much you can do except take a bath or shower together after making love!

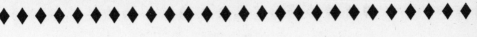

Lochia

→ Lochia is the vaginal discharge that occurs after you give birth.
→ Think of lochia as your body cleaning itself, the uterus shedding what it no longer needs.
→ If you are accustomed to lovemaking when you have your period, this will be similar.

Pain during sex

→ Pain can occur at the vaginal opening or inside the vagina.
→ Your perineum (the area between your anus and vagina) may be sore due to bruising or tears.
→ Even women who have had cesarean deliveries can have some discomfort during sex.
→ It may be a good idea for the woman to be on top during lovemaking so that she can control the amount of penetration.
→ Give yourself time to heal. Let your partner know how your body is feeling so he'll understand.

When can we have sex again?

→ Many doctors suggest waiting for six weeks after childbirth.
→ A six-week wait may be too long for many couples.
→ If you had no tears and no episiotomy there is no reason not to resume within three weeks.
→ Ask your doctor about resuming sex sooner: if you feel his or her recommendation is too conservative, get another doctor's opinion.
→ A good way to judge whether your body is ready is when the lochia disappears and/or when your episiotomy incision has healed.

7.
Bits and Pieces

Miscellaneous Advice
for the Wait

CHOOSING
A PEDIATRICIAN

When to start looking

* You'll want to choose a pediatrician before the baby is born.
* Some pediatricians will meet with you and your partner without charge when you are pregnant.
* If you choose a pediatrician beforehand, the hospital notifies him as soon as the baby is born.
* This means your own pediatrician examines the baby instead of a doctor from the hospital staff.

WHAT TO LOOK FOR
WHEN CHOOSING YOUR PEDIATRICIAN

The office location — It helps to live close to the office if you have to bring a sick child to the doctor.

House calls — Pediatricians are just about the only doctors who sometimes make house calls. Ask whether the doctor does, and under what circumstances.

How busy is the practice? — You shouldn't have to call too far ahead for an appointment. Can they see the baby quickly in an emergency?

Is it a group practice? — If your doctor shares the practice with one or more doctors, will your child see a different doctor each time? (You'll probably want to develop a relationship with the pediatrician you choose.)

The doctor's personality — Do you (and your mate) feel at ease with him or her? Does she or he have a sense of humor? Seem warm toward children? Is she or he patronizing toward you or respectful?

The doctor's style of child rearing — The doctor's attitude will affect you: find out whether he or she prefers a rigid style or has a more loose and unstructured attitude. There's no "right" way to be a parent, but it's better to choose a pediatrician with attitudes similar to your own.

Attitudes about feeding the baby — It helps if a doctor is open-minded about how an infant is fed. Whether you decide to breast-feed, bottle-feed, or a combination, you'll probably need encouragement at some point.

Attitudes toward working mothers — If you'll be working when your baby is small a doctor's disapproval can undermine your self-confidence as a mother.

Circumcision — This is a decision you should discuss with your pediatrician before the baby is born. A doctor can give you his opinion and the pros and cons, but if you have a strong opinion either way, you should find a doctor who supports your decision.

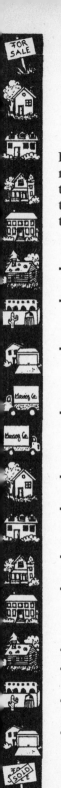

MOVING: IS IT WORTH IT?

It's natural to think about moving when you're expecting a new member of the family. There are choices to make about whether to move and how to make it easier on yourselves if you decide to. Knowing that you have a choice makes you feel in control of the situation. This automatically relieves some pressure.

Reasons not to move when pregnant

→ Moving involves a lot of physical and emotional demands: it's a big life change.

→ Why put yourself through that kind of strain if you don't have to? Being pregnant already presents you with plenty of adjustments you have to make.

→ The stress of moving multiplied by the physical and emotional demands of pregnancy ... and the changes you have to go through in pregnancy ... are increased by the demands of moving (it's sort of like 2 + 2 = 10!)

→ Moving to a new geographical area—even if it's only a different neighborhood—requires even more because you have to find your way around, make personal connections, establish new services.

→ You don't have the energy or stamina you had before pregnancy to cope with the physical demands of moving.

→ The physical complaints of pregnancy are going to be aggravated by moving. And problems like nausea and fatigue can make it more difficult to plan and carry out a move.

→ The first trimester is when a pregnancy is at risk for miscarriage; moving at that time creates unnecessary stress.

→ In the first trimester, as you get bigger, it becomes harder to get around easily.

Questions to ask before moving

"Can I afford it?"

→ Does a larger space mean taking on too heavy a financial burden?

→ Moving usually leaves you with less money to spend: can you cope with that?

→ Will these pressures genuinely be offset by the convenience of more space or a better family neighborhood?

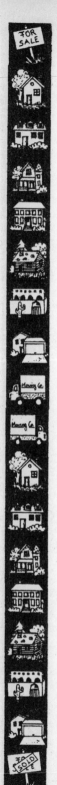

"Do I have enough time for all the demands?"
→ First there is hunting for the house or apartment.
→ Then you have to organize the paperwork if you're buying.
→ Next you need to organize your belongings for the move.
→ Finally there are the demands of settling into a new place.

"Do I have the energy?"
→ Packing and unpacking take a lot of strength, even if you get help.
→ You have to be on your feet a lot and do lifting and carrying.
→ In the first trimester you may feel sleepy and/or nauseated.
→ In the last trimester you may tire easily and/or be too big to get around easily.
→ It's not advisable to lift heavy objects as your due date gets closer.

"Will the actual work of moving create marital discord?"
→ Will your mate realistically be able to pitch in to the extent you expect or need?
→ If you do most of the work, will your mate feel guilty that he can't do his "fair share"—or irritated that he's expected to?
→ Will you be resentful that he hasn't done more?

"What about waiting a year?"
→ An infant doesn't require much space until he is walking around.
→ Could you handle the demands of moving better a year from now?
→ Being pregnant takes more out of you than you may realize; a year from now your body will probably have more stamina.

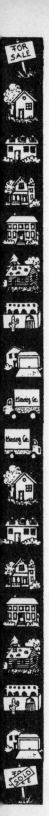
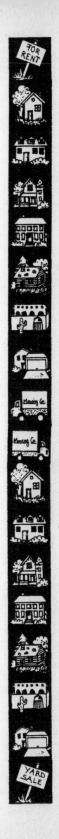

SURVIVAL RULES FOR MOVING
WHILE PREGNANT

❖ DO NOT LIFT OR PUSH heavy objects. You can hurt yourself now because pregnancy hormones affect your ligaments and muscles.

❖ DO NOT TRY TO BE SUPERWOMAN and do everything all
at once.

❖ DO NOT EXHAUST YOURSELF. You simply don't have the
energy or stamina you did before pregnancy. It's also
harder to bounce back when you're pregnant.

❖ DO NOT CLIMB UP ON THINGS. Stay off ladders, step
stools, windowsills, etc. Your sense of balance is off, especially as your belly gets bigger.

❖ DON'T TRY TO DO IT ALONE. Get help whenever and
from whomever you can, paid or unpaid. Ask friends or
relatives: if none is around, pay a handyman or neighborhood teenager to help organize things before the professional movers come in.

❖ DON'T TRY TO SAVE MONEY ON SERVICES. Pay the
movers (or others, see above) to do as much packing and
unpacking as possible. It is money well spent.

TRAVELING DURING PREGNANCY

* Traveling does not cause miscarriage, premature labor, or other complications—but they could be more frightening or inconvenient if you were away from home.
* Check with your obstetrician before planning a trip, just to be safe.
* If you take a trip of any distance at any time during pregnancy, your obstetrician should give you the name of a doctor where you're going, just in case.

CONSULT YOUR DOCTOR BEFORE TRAVELING IF . . .

❖ Your pregnancy is high-risk (high blood pressure, diabetes, or other complications).

❖ You have a history of miscarriage or premature labor.

❖ You're in the first trimester (some doctors recommend against making a long or strenuous trip because the possibility of miscarriage is highest now).

❖ You're in the last six weeks of pregnancy. The doctor will probably recommend not going more than fifty miles from home.

Pregnant travel tips

→ You're more prone to motion sickness now so don't travel on an empty stomach.
→ Eat light snacks; avoid big portions or food that's rich, fried, or otherwise indigestible.
→ Bring nutritious snacks with you on any length trip, even a day's outing. You never know when you'll get hungry; it's better to have protein bars, carrot sticks, or raisins than to find nothing but a doughnut shop to satisfy your appetite!

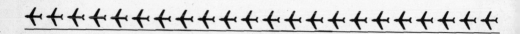

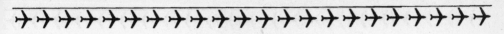

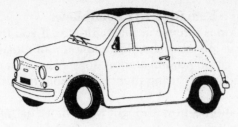

Car travel

→ Fasten your seat belt, using the shoulder harness too.
  - Seat belts may seem uncomfortable but they can reduce injuries and save your life.
  - Buckle it low, below your belly, across your pelvis.
→ It may not seem like it, but sitting in a car can be tiring; limit yourself to a maximum of three hundred miles a day.
→ Stop and get out at least every one hundred miles (or two hours of driving) to walk around for your circulation.
→ You can do the driving while you're pregnant ... as long as you fit behind the wheel!

Air travel

→ Many airlines have rules about pregnant passengers: check beforehand if you need documentation like a doctor's note.
→ Do not fly in a small private plane with an unpressurized cabin: it can reduce the oxygen reaching your baby.
→ If you're prone to air sickness sit over the wings or toward the front: you'll feel less of the plane's motion.
→ Go to the bathroom before takeoff. You need to urinate more frequently now and there may be a delay in takeoff or the seat belt sign may stay on a long time.
→ Drink plenty of liquids: air travel makes all passengers dehydrated and you're especially vulnerable.
→ Fasten your seat belt below your belly, across the pelvis.
→ If it's a long trip get up at least every two hours to stretch your legs and insure good circulation.
→ Don't wear constricting clothing, especially panty-hose or knee-high socks that could cut off your circulation.
→ Choose roomy shoes. *Everyone's* feet swell on a long plane trip; it's even more true during pregnancy.
→ Flying isn't a good idea after the seventh month; although it does not cause labor, the chance of going into labor increases as your due date approaches.

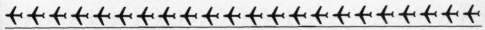

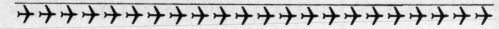

Radiation risk in airplanes

→ Cosmic radiation is intense at high altitudes. If you fly frequently you can absorb a significant amount of radiation.

→ The Federal Aviation Administration doesn't have an up-to-date safe level of radiation during flight, according to radiation experts.

→ Low-level radiation is now thought to be more harmful than was previously believed.

→ Extreme doses of radiation in flight can increase the risk of birth defects in the developing baby.

    • Long-term effects of significant prenatal radiation are not yet known.

    • One result can be a possible loss of IQ or school performance.

→ The "mSv" (millisievert) is the unit that indicates the quantity and intensity of radiation exposure.

→ Occupationally exposed people like flight attendants take note:

    • In the United States 50 mSv is considered a tolerable limit.

    • The acceptable limit for European employees in similar jobs is 15 mSv.

    • For comparison, a chest X-ray exposes your body to 0.1 mSv.

→ The recommended annual limit of radiation for all travelers is 1 mSv.

    • Below are the estimated doses of radiation for flying round-trip between various cities.

    • Multiply the dose of radiation by the number of times you fly that route or a similar one.

ROUTE	DOSE IN mSv
NY/Tokyo; NY/Athens	0.20
LA/London	0.16
Chicago/London; LA/Tokyo	0.12
Dallas/London; NY/London	0.10
NY/Seattle; NY/Lisbon	0.08
Chicago/San Francisco	0.06
Washington, DC/LA; Honolulu/LA	0.05
Chicago/NY; Minneapolis/NY	0.02

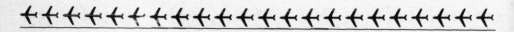

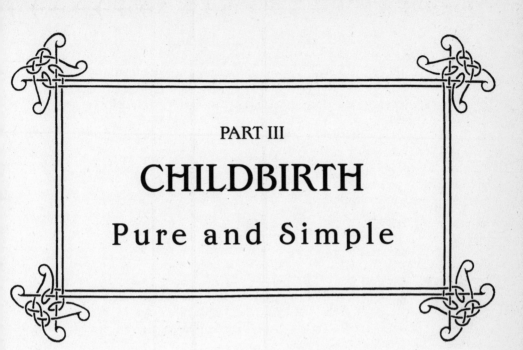

PART III

CHILDBIRTH

Pure and Simple

8.

Choices in Childbirth

When, Where, and How

There are a variety of settings in which to give
birth and some choice in the professionals you
can choose to support and guide you through
your baby's birth. By exercising the freedom
to choose, you can personalize your birth
experience.

CHOOSING A DOCTOR

Before interviewing obstetricians you should talk to friends and friends of friends about their experiences; that's an efficient way to "vet out" a doctor. (Ask someone who's had a baby within the last five years; if it's been much longer than that a doctor may have changed techniques, attitude, or partners).

Questions for Friends About Their Doctor

"During prenatal care did the doctor and/or office staff make time to answer your questions and respond to your concerns?"

"During labor when did the doctor arrive and how long did s/he stay?"

"Once you were in labor, what was the doctor's attitude to Lamaze? To having medication?"

"Did you get the support, compassion, or medical intervention you felt you needed?"

"What would be your main complaint, if any, about the doctor?"

"Would you [did you] have another baby with the same doctor? And why?"

Questions to Ask a Father

"How would you rate the doctor's attitude and supportiveness toward you during prenatal care?"

"How was his/her bedside manner during office visits and labor?"

"What about the way the doctor handled any problems?"

"What was the doctor's attitude toward your involvement or lack of it in the childbirth experience?"

"Did you have any interaction with the doctor after delivery?"

Questions for the Doctor

- Once you've found a doctor, the *way* you ask questions is important.
- Recognize that doctors are usually deferred to: that's the nature of being a doctor.
- Be polite but get the information you need to make an informed decision.
- Ask questions about your greatest concerns, choosing a few key points rather than a barrage of demands.

"Do many of your patients take childbirth classes? What percentage of them wind up giving birth without medication?"

"Do the other doctors in your practice share your views on most aspects of childbirth? When would I get to meet them?"

"How often do you induce labor? Under what circumstances?"

"I'm a worrywart and might have a lot of neurotic questions during my pregnancy. Do you have a time of day set aside for those kinds of phone calls or do you have a nurse I could call when I need answers?"

"If a cesarean is necessary, how do you feel about the father being present?"

"Would you consider eliminating any of the routine hospital procedures for labor and delivery?"

"Do you always do an episiotomy?"

Questions for the Doctor's Staff

You can ask these questions on the telephone or in person.

Office visits

"How often are office visits scheduled?"

"How many appointments do you book per hour?" (or "How much time do you allow for each visit?")

"What tests are standard?"

Payment

"What is the fee?"

"When is full payment required?"

"What does it cover?"

"What would be extra?"

Hospital affiliation

"Does the doctor use more than one hospital?"

"If so, what are the differences between them?"

"Where have women seemed to have the better birth experience?"

Labor and delivery

"When does the doctor usually arrive at the hospital?"

"If labor is slow does the doctor go back to the office and return later?"

"What is the likelihood that another doctor in the practice will deliver my baby?"

Diet

"What recommendations do you make about nutrition and weight gain?"

Breast-feeding

"Do you have a support system for breast-feeding?"

"Do you loan videos, have a nurse specializing in breast-feeding, or have a telephone 'hotline' for help?"

CHOOSING A HOSPITAL

Types of hospitals

CATHOLIC HOSPITALS

- Catholic hospitals account for one third of hospital beds in the United States.
- They usually have restrictive policies.
- Ask questions beforehand about any topics that concern you.

TEACHING HOSPITALS

- Teaching hospitals have the best medical facilities.
- Doctors at teaching hospitals see more births and more complicated births, so they are better equipped to handle problems.
- There will be many interns and residents observing in a teaching hospital.

SMALL COMMUNITY HOSPITAL

- This type of hospital can be more flexible.
- You may be able to arrange a more individualized childbirth.
- They will probably lack the costly equipment found in a teaching hospital.

FAMILY-CENTERED MATERNITY CARE

- Individualized care offered by more progressive hospitals.
- Certain choices associated with family-centered care include:
    - Leboyer delivery
    - Breast-feeding on the delivery table
    - Nonseparation of parents and baby
    - Early discharge

Things to find out about hospital policies

BREAST-FEEDING

- Is nursing encouraged immediately after birth on the delivery table?

- Do they routinely give newborns a bottle of glucose and water in the nursery? (A bottle can make breast-feeding more difficult because the baby is satisfied by the sugar water that was easier to suck from a rubber nipple.)
- Is a baby allowed to breast-feed on demand?

[NOTE:"On demand" means that your baby is brought to you (if you are separated) whenever she or he cries. Otherwise, the baby could be on an every-four-hour schedule imposed by the hospital.]

Miscellaneous hospital policies

Early discharge
- If birth is unmedicated you can leave the hospital six to twenty-four hours after birth.
- Advantage is lower hospital bills and recovery in the comfort and privacy of your own home.

Photographs and tape recording
- Often forbidden in many large hospitals.
- If permitted, is a release form required when you preregister?
- Is flash equipment banned?
- If there are no rules against photos, do you still require the doctor's consent?

Prenatal education classes
- What percentage of women who give birth at the hospital have had childbirth preparation?
- This indicates whether the staff is familiar with and supportive of Lamaze.

Preregistration
- Saves time and aggravation to be already registered when you arrive in labor.
- How much money is required on admittance and discharge? (So you can come prepared.)
- If they don't offer preregistration, can you fill out just the important forms on arrival and do the rest later?

Rooming-in
- Can you keep your baby in your room with you?
- Do you have the choice of having the baby with you during the day but sending him back to the nursery at night?
- Advantages: You can learn your baby's needs from birth. Encourages bonding and adjusting to each other.

Enema	■ Given routinely to women in early labor.
	■ Empties lower bowel to give the baby as much room as possible.
	■ The embarrassment of pushing out fecal matter may inhibit some women from pushing.
	■ An enema can cause strong contractions.
	■ If you have not eaten much before the beginning of labor or if you have had a bowel movement fairly recently, you may not want to have an enema.
Intravenous drip (IV)	■ An IV of glucose and water is often given to women in labor to provide fluids and energy.
	■ An IV can be restricting and limits your movements.
	■ If your doctor insists on using an IV he may wait until delivery before inserting it, giving you hours of labor beforehand without it.
Shaving	■ It is not medically necessary to shave your pubic hair before delivery.
	■ It was originally done to avoid infection, but studies show that shaving can increase infection.
	■ Shaving facilitates the episiotomy repair for the doctor.
	■ One option is to request a "mini prep," which means that instead of your entire pubic area's being shaved, it will be only the lips of the vagina.

COPING WITH THE HOSPITAL

* Hospitals can be intimidating and rigid.
* Your expectations for a wonderful personalized birth experience may be unrealistic.
* The very atmosphere of a hospital can create anxiety.
* It's good to know what to expect and how to deal with hospital staff in order to have the best experience.

Avoiding routine procedures
→ Find out hospital policies ahead of time.
→ Recognize that if you sidestep routines you take on the responsibility for anything that goes wrong.
→ Get a note from your obstetrician stating which routines can be eliminated.
→ Get a note from your pediatrician stating which routines you and the doctor agree need not be performed with your baby.

Lamaze and the hospital staff
→ Be sure to tell the hospital staff that you've taken childbirth preparation.
→ Don't respond to any staff interruptions during a contraction.
→ Afterward explain your need to concentrate: you will be able to interact *between* contractions.
→ Do not let any staff member's attitude aggravate you. Getting upset is going to interfere with your labor and childbirth experience.
→ Let hospital personnel know you are educated about childbirth and determined to do your best to stay on top of the situation with your training.

ALTERNATIVE BIRTHING CENTERS
(ABCs)

→ ABCs are available in a limited number of hospitals across the country.

→ A homelike environment is created within the hospital where a woman can deliver almost as if she were at home.

→ Only "low-risk" women with no indications of potential problems have the option of using an ABC.

→ There are no *routine* drugs or medical intervention (options are available once you're in labor but they're your choice).

→ Siblings are allowed to attend the birth (with an adult escort).

→ You have the option of inviting friends (although space is usually limited).

→ You can choose any position for labor and delivery that suits you.

→ You can leave the hospital within six to twenty-four hours after an unmedicated birth if everything's normal with you and the baby.

→ Many hospitals have incorporated the intentions of an ABC by upgrading the quality of the labor and delivery areas, redesigning them as multipurpose birthing rooms.

→ Hospitals now view ABC as more of a concept than a specific place.

THE FETAL HEART MONITOR (FHM)

Controversy continues about the FHM. Some hail it as the greatest advance in the history of maternity care; others attack it as inaccurate and dehumanizing. It is important to educate yourself about fetal monitoring so you can be informed and objective if you have to decide when to use it during childbirth.

How the fetal monitor works
→ Two wide straps are placed around your stomach; one records your uterine contractions, the other charts the baby's heart rate.
→ You must lie quite still to avoid false results from your movements.
→ An internal monitor can replace the lower strap for more accurate results.
→ The internal monitor is either a screw or clip electrode. It is inserted through your vagina (once your cervix is dilated to at least one to two centimeters). It is attached to your baby's scalp or inserted just under her skin.
→ Some hospitals use the internal monitor whenever a woman's membranes have broken; others wait until fetal distress has been detected with external monitoring.

What happens if the FHM shows fetal distress?
→ If there is a distress pattern the staff will reposition you, usually turning you on your side.
→ The staff will increase your blood pressure by giving you an IV and administering oxygen with a face mask.
→ Fetal scalp sampling is performed to determine whether distress suggested by the FHM is accurate.
  ▸ Scalp sampling is done by making a tiny prick in the baby's presenting part (usually the head).
  ▸ The blood is examined for its concentration of oxygen, carbon dioxide, and pH.
  ▸ It is hoped that the newest internal monitors will be so accurate that blood analysis will not be as frequent.
→ As a rule of thumb, if a normal heart rate pattern cannot be restored in a previously healthy baby within half an hour, a cesarean section is performed.

LEBOYER DELIVERY

Developed by a French doctor who aimed to reduce the trauma of labor and delivery experienced by the newborn, Leboyer delivery focuses attention on the baby, encouraging awareness of her. Many hospitals offer variations on these themes.

Leboyer's recommendations for birth

→ Dim, indirect lighting (more comfortable for the newborn's sensitive eyes).

→ A warmer delivery room temperature (adjusted to the comfort of the *baby*, not the adults).

→ Immediate positioning of the newborn on the mother's stomach and minimal blanketing of the newborn (more skin-to-skin contact to enhance maternal-infant bonding).

→ A minimum of loud noise and talk (although a newborn's ears are probably filled with fluid at birth, so sounds are naturally softened).

→ Gentle handling of the baby.

→ Delay severing the umbilical cord until pulsation has stopped.

→ Placing the newborn in a tub of warm water (in America the father gives the bath).

Objections to Leboyer techniques

→ The bath can chill the baby, who doesn't yet have an efficient system to maintain body heat.

→ Some doctors think the shock of the environment stimulates the newborn's breathing—that nature intended him to leave the watery womb and make an abrupt transition.

→ Some women do not want to hand the baby over for a bath if they have already begun breast-feeding and the baby is content.

→ The bath may interfere with bonding if it is imposed routinely without considering if it's an interruption.

FRIENDS AND FAMILY ATTENDING THE BIRTH

Sharing the birth with guests

→ In maternity center births and alternative birthing rooms (ABCs) in hospitals it's usually an option to have guests.

→ Emotional support is important during childbirth; being surrounded by friends can give you that feeling.

→ Guests should probably not arrive until you are well established in labor.

→ Outsiders' presence and comments might make you feel tense and slow the progress of early labor.

→ Discuss beforehand your preferences:

  ❧ Any particular behavior or reactions you want to request or discourage.

  ❧ Reserve the option to ask people to leave at any time during the birth.

→ If there are children present there should be one adult per child to supervise and entertain them.

CHILDBIRTH CLASSES

How childbirth techniques work
→ Childbirth classes train you so that relaxation becomes a built-in response.
→ Taking childbirth classes can shorten the length of labor and make it more manageable.
→ One of the most useful things you learn is to take labor one step at a time, dealing with each contraction as it happens without worrying about what's ahead.

Coping with pain
→ Childbirth education prepares you to control the pain of labor.
→ How much pain you'll have is partially determined by whether you have had childbirth training and how committed you are.
→ Your menstrual history is an indicator of pain during childbirth: women with acute cramping at the beginning of their periods tend to have more pain during childbirth.

Finding a childbirth class
→ To find a class in your area ask your friends or your obstetrician.
→ Choosing a class is mostly a matter of finding a teacher whose style and personality make you feel comfortable.
→ Most teachers will give you a class outline and let you sit in on one of their classes before signing up.
→ A good size class is usually eight to ten couples.
→ Classes usually start in your seventh month and meet once a week for six to ten weeks.
→ Most classes are basically the same, although there are slight differences in the type of breathing they teach.
→ The Lamaze method is the most well known—yet originally it did not include the husband as coach (an idea initiated by Dr. Robert Bradley of the "Bradley Method").
→ The differences are usually over how much the teacher encourages drug-free birth.

The father's involvement

→ Including the father is one of the important benefits of childbirth classes.

→ It gives you an opportunity to work as a team, learning to trust each other totally.

→ Some men are reluctant to start classes but as they begin to see their role during labor they usually become more relaxed and confident.

THE COACH WHO ISN'T YOUR HUSBAND

There are various reasons your partner may not coach you.

→ It's not advisable to coerce or otherwise pressure your husband if he doesn't want to be with you through childbirth.

→ If you're a single mother you can view finding a childbirth coach as good practice for the resourcefulness that parenting alone will demand of you!

→ Your "significant other" can be a close friend; your mother, sister, or other relative; or even a male friend if your friendship is that intimate.

→ Don't put yourself on the defensive in childbirth class (or labor) by explaining why your coach isn't your husband! It's no one else's business and is irrelevant to the main event.

→ Don't lose sight of what matters! The important thing is that you have someone to practice with who can then guide you through your child's birth.

UNDERWATER BIRTH

→ There is a fad going around for delivering babies into a tub of water, which is potentially dangerous.
  - Fortunately, this gimmick is not widespread, but it still represents a fatal danger to the innocent victims.
  - No mammal on earth goes into the water to deliver its young, except whales . . . which live in the water, of course.
→ The justification for underwater birth:
  - It allows the newborn to go from one liquid environment to another.
  - The theory is that this will lessen the trauma of birth.
→ Birth is *supposed* to be a shock to a baby's system!
  - Your newborn has to make the critical adjustment from life inside your uterus to existence in the outside world.
  - The baby's health and survival depend on how well s/he makes this transition.
→ Once the placenta separates, the baby is on her own.
  - The baby's lungs must supply oxygen the moment the placenta—the intrauterine supply—is cut off.
  - With a baby born underwater there's no way to tell when the placenta has separated; the baby may take water into her lungs instead of air.
  - The baby will drown if she breathes in water—this has happened to people experimenting with underwater birthing.
→ How can you do an Apgar test underwater?
  - The first few minutes of the baby's life are critical in assessing how s/he's adjusting to life "on the outside."
  - The point of the Apgar test is to monitor a baby's responses: s/he can get immediate help if there are difficulties.
  - There is no way to make this judgment about a baby who is underwater.
→ Why would any parents be willing to take this life-threatening risk for their baby?

9.
The Emotional Aspects of Childbirth

Pregnancy is a time when a woman's feelings about herself and her life can feel as though they're thrown up into the air like a handful of confetti! Understanding your emotions—and those of your partner—at this turning point in your life can make going through these changes easier and more interesting.

BECOMING A MOTHER

The responsibilities of becoming a mother can be exhausting and overwhelming. You may want to get out and work or you may have to work for economic reasons. But there are still the dishes to do, the baby to feed, and a husband to think about!

A feeling of motherhood
→ Not everyone feels an instant bond with her child.
→ Don't feel guilty if it takes some time to get used to the idea of being a mother.
→ Feelings of loving warmth and protectiveness will grow with time.

Fear of incompetence
→ Every mom feels uneasy at first. By trial and error you'll figure things out.
→ If you don't know something, ask a friend for help or read a baby-care book.
→ Before long it will all become second-nature to you.

Don't try to be a supermom.
→ Accept yourself for what you do and do not like about baby-tending. Not everyone gets as kick out of changing diapers!
→ It is okay to be annoyed that you have to get up during the night for feedings.

Tune out everyone else's theories.
→ Other people may think they know what is "right" but everyone is different.
→ Get whatever facts you need and then trust your own instincts and judgment.

FEARS AND DOUBTS
ABOUT MOTHERHOOD

Apprehensions about motherhood are to be expected.
→ There are questions everyone asks.
→ "Do I want to give up so much to become a mother?" "Will I be any good at it?" "Will my marriage adjust?"

Feeling uncomfortable about being a caretaker is normal.
→ If you doubt your ability to take care of the baby, just think about the many things you have taken care of in the past: a sick husband, your siblings, older relatives, plants, pets, etc.

Don't worry if you don't have a "maternal instinct" right away.
→ Lots of women take time to warm up to their babies; not every mother feels immediate adoration for the newborn.
→ Give yourself time; love will grow.
→ Mothering is a skill you learn by tuning in to your baby and letting her responses guide you.

It's normal to have doubts about baby care.
→ Every woman has to do "on-the-job-training" to acquire the skills for infant care.
→ No one "just naturally" knows how to handle bathing, nail-clipping, crying fits, etc.
→ A mother is something you learn how to be, day by day.

Worries about feeling bored or trapped are realistic.
→ Caring for a baby is not totally enjoyable.
→ If you're concerned about feelings of isolation or frustrated by new motherhood you may just be more honest about motherhood than other people.

Negative thoughts about parenting make you feel guilty.
→ Instead of worrying why other mothers don't complain, feel good that you're facing the realistic burdens of parenting.
→ Anxiety and stress are part of motherhood; recognizing this is a healthy part of preparation for your new life.

Admitting doubts, fears, and resentments is important.

→ Hiding negative feelings (as many new mothers do) can make them seem worse than they are and create tension and pressure.

→ Bad feelings are nothing to be ashamed of—releasing them allows you to grow more gracefully into motherhood.

YOUR RELATIONSHIP WITH YOUR MOTHER

Feelings about your own upbringing influence what you will be like as a mother.

→ The mothering you got can inspire you to re-create your childhood or to improve on the mothering you got.

→ In all likelihood you'll be more like your mother than you expect. This is true even for women who want to be very different!

Your mother's style of mothering may not be yours.

→ There may be aspects of your mother's personality that make you want to embrace the opposite style of parenting.

→ You may have complicated feelings about your experiences with her that are going to influence you as a parent more than you realize.

What's your current relationship with your mother?

→ Whether you're close or estranged, your having a baby will change your attitudes toward each other.

→ A baby can signal a new era of understanding, forgiveness, and closeness.

Will you win your mother's love or approval with a grandchild?

→ If you feel your mother didn't love you (or loved your sibling more) your baby may represent a way to get your mother's affection now. If this sounds like something that might be affecting you subconsciously, it's worth thinking about.

THE SUPERMOM SYNDROME

> ## MISTAKEN BELIEFS OF A SUPERMOM
>
> ✤ You can never disappoint anyone or let them down.
> ✤ You are constantly giving, doing, planning.
> ✤ You can protect your child from bad experiences.
> ✤ You can do it all, be everything for everyone.
> ✤ You take total responsibility for your child's experience of life.
> ✤ If your child isn't perfectly well adjusted, it's your fault.

→ Idealized images of motherhood make it hard to be a real mother in the real world. Saintly stereotypes of mothers form our ideas of what a mother should be like: generous, kind, patient, putting others first, and fulfilled by dedicating her life to her children.

→ A supermom has to be everything for everyone. Believing that sets you up for unrealistic expectations of yourself (with the likelihood of frequently feeling guilty or like a failure!).

→ Society glorifies motherhood. The myth is that a mother is supposed to be all-loving and all-giving . . . without ambition for herself . . . never giving in to fatigue, anger, or resentment. (Who wouldn't be nervous about new motherhood with that image to live up to?)

To guard against becoming a supermom, say:

→ "I'm just an ordinary human being, like everyone else."

→ "Twenty-four hours is the maximum number for any day—and there's only so much I can get done."

→ "Are the goals I'm setting realistic—or could any of them be described as compulsive or neurotic?"

→ "Who else can do this task? Does it need to be done at all?"

→ "I cannot do everything 'to the max': be a loving, compassionate wife *AND* have a satisfying career *AND* give the baby the time and affection he needs *AND* run a household that's shipshape. I'm only human. *Really!*"

FATIGUE

- Fatigue is common: continue taking your iron pills for six weeks after childbirth.
- Because the baby has no conception of day and night, you can expect to get limited sleep during the first six to eight weeks after birth.
- Some women find it is many months (even a full year) before they sleep well again after the birth of their child.

Ways to avoid a fatigue cycle
→ Good nutrition helps combat fatigue.
→ Don't eat heavily or drink caffeine or other stimulating drinks before you to go bed.
→ Half an hour before "bedtime" get into bed with warm milk and read, watch TV, or listen to music.
→ Take naps when the baby naps.

ISOLATION

- Isolation is a common problem for new mothers.
- You may find yourself home alone for eight hours or more without adult conversation.
- This can cause depression.
→ Finding friends who have recent experience with babies can provide emotional support. If you aren't close to anyone with small children try to find organizations of parents or get together with women from your childbirth class.
→ Your mother can be a wonderful source of support if you have a good relationship.
→ It is important to get away from the confines of your house, either with or without the baby, for some period of time every day.

GETTING HELP AT HOME

→ It is important to rest after the baby is born.
→ The time you spend with your baby is most important: you will benefit from having help running the house.
→ *Interview* before the baby is born.
→ If you are going to get professional help, ask friends whether they used anyone they would recommend, or contact a domestic employment agency.
→ Check recent references on *anyone* you're considering.

Choices in childcare

A TRAINED BABY NURSE

● If you are ill at ease taking care of a newborn, a professional baby nurse can show you how everything should be done.
● Be aware that they won't do housework or cooking—and they can be expensive, besides.

A PRACTICAL NURSE OR PROFESSIONAL BABY-SITTER

She will do light housework, some cooking, and also look after the baby and show you the ropes.

RELATIVES

● Depending on the relationship you have with your mother or mother-in-law you may find relatives a great help or a pain in the neck.
● If you have doubts you might want to wait until the baby is two or three months old. By then you'll be in a routine and less vulnerable to feeling dominated.

MOOD SWINGS

- Moodiness affects all pregnant women at one time or another.
- You may have rapidly shifting moods in response to situations that wouldn't usually trigger such extreme reactions.
- Unexplained crying, emotional outbursts, and attacks of anxiety are not uncommon.
- You may also forget where you put things, forget appointments, mix up information, drop things, and generally walk around in a daze.
- This can be a result of hormonal changes along with focusing all your attention inward on yourself and the pregnancy.

Reasons for moodiness

HORMONAL CHANGES

Your body is producing large amounts of progesterone, which has a depressant effect on the central nervous system.

PMS

If you suffered from premenstrual syndrome before, be prepared for mood swings now. If you got cranky or weepy before your period that same sensitivity to hormones will probably affect you during pregnancy.

BODY-IMAGE CHANGES

Your dramatically changing body may affect your self-esteem or image of yourself.

IDENTITY ISSUES

You're about to change your role in life. This is a big one to deal with.

Ambivalence About Pregnancy and Motherhood

Mixed feelings about having a baby and becoming a parent can make you feel confused or guilty.

Unresolved or Unacknowledged Feelings

Denying what's going on inside can cause moodiness.

Fear About Childbirth or Parenting

Feeling frightened (and not knowing the feelings are normal) can lead to mood swings.

How to Handle Mood Swings

✤ Don't suppress emotions: bottled-up feelings can grow larger and surface in unpredictable ways.

✤ Don't be unrealistic in expectations of yourself: you have real issues to worry about, so don't expect to resolve conflicts or overcome fears completely.

✤ Try to roll with the feelings: don't fight your emotions or try to swallow them. "Resistance creates persistence": don't fight mood swings and they'll roll off your back more easily.

✤ Don't try to figure out the "deeper meaning" of your moods. (They probably don't have any deep meaning!) You'll only prolong the problem if you make a big deal asking *"Why?"* every time you have a down period. Try to view the slumps as one end of the mood spectrum, with an upswing on the way.

✤ Recognize that depression, anxiety, and confusion occur in even the most happy pregnancies.

COPING WITH STRESS

→ During pregnancy you can be more vulnerable to outside stresses.

→ Stress may hit you harder now.

→ You may not bounce back from problems as easily as you did before pregnancy.

→ Normal everyday problems may seem more difficult to handle.

→ If you can *accept* that things just seem rougher now, it can help you roll with the punches.

→ Typical causes of stress that can affect people at any time, but can appear worse during pregnancy, are listed below:

PROBLEMS THAT CAN APPEAR BIGGER NOW

❖ Tension in your marriage

❖ Health problems: yours and anyone's in your family

❖ Your financial situation

❖ Moving to a new home

❖ Moving to a new geographic area

❖ Changing or ending a job

→ The box opposite has symptoms that may be due to a high level of stress.

→ These can also be signs of a woman unconsciously rejecting her pregnancy.

→ Getting help during pregnancy can nip problems in the bud and keep issues from becoming larger and more overwhelming.

→ Talking to a therapist before the baby arrives can help you resolve problems before the exhaustion and distraction of early motherhood interferes with clear thinking.

→ If you are aware you're under stress and have any of the symptoms opposite, consider getting professional help now.

WARNING SIGNS OF
REACTIONS TO STRESS

+ Preoccupation with your physical appearance
+ Negative perception of yourself
+ Excessive physical complaints
+ No emotional reaction when the baby moves inside you
+ No effort in the last trimester to prepare the baby's room or clothing

FEARS, WORRIES, AND ANXIETIES

THINGS YOU MAY BE WORRIED ABOUT

The Anxiety	Dealing with It
Will the baby be normal?	Get appropriate tests, then let it go.
I drank before knowing I was pregnant.	It takes more than a few drinks to cause defects in most cases.
I ate foods I didn't know were unhealthy early in pregnancy.	Eat extra-well now.
Loss of freedom	Find a more positive description of motherhood.
Changes in lifestyle	View change as an adventure, a challenge.
Fear of being an inadequate mother	Mothering is something learned: there are no grades!
Inability to care for baby	Everybody has to learn the skills: mistakes are okay.
Self-doubt about being emotionally equipped for motherhood	You'll grow into it.
Loss of attractiveness	Believe pregnancy is beautiful and so will those around you.
Labor and delivery	You'll do the best you can—and that will be good enough.
General angst and anxiety	Talk out feelings to discover specific concerns.

Being worried is normal!
→ Being pregnant and facing parenthood mean many reasons to worry for anyone expecting. You're not alone!
→ Many of your concerns are probably justified: a new baby is a big deal in anyone's life.
→ Your partner may share many of your concerns; the baby's father's feelings are on page 196.

→ Dealing with these fears is part of preparing to be a parent. Think of it as a "dry run" for what it will feel like the first time your baby rides a tricycle or takes the school bus!

→ Don't deny your feelings—it's healthy to deal with emotions. If you brush off fears as unimportant or silly, the emotions can surface later . . . in a way and at a place where you least expect them.

POSTPARTUM DEPRESSION

"Baby blues," or postpartum depression, affects many women. It usually last one to seven days and is marked by tearfulness, anxiety, depression, restlessness, and irritability.

REASONS FOR POSTPARTUM DEPRESSION

Hormones

Hormone adjustment can cause this emotional unpleasantness.

Lowered thyroid function

If you are feeling low for more than a few days after the baby's birth you should have your thyroid level checked.

Your personality

How you generally deal with stress can influence your feelings about motherhood. If you're an anxious person you're more likely to be upset by your new responsibilities.

What is postpartum depression?
- Also called PPD, it is the temporary mental imbalance that many women experience after childbirth.
- It is usually the result of changes in hormones and brain chemicals.

When does it happen?
- PPD usually happens in the first three weeks after childbirth.
- The depression can range from mild blues to psychosis (with severe mood swings and hallucinations).

What causes it?
- The hormonal changes after the baby is born are the central reason for PPD.
- The huge drop in hormone levels affects your mental state.

Who gets PPD?
- Almost all women experience some symptoms of what are also called "baby blues."

- A smaller group of women have a more serious and longer emotional reaction after childbirth.
- PPD can affect any woman: strong, well-adjusted ones as easily as nervous, neurotic ones.

PPD is almost impossible to predict.

- There are a few factors that can make a new mother more vulnerable to PPD (see box below).
- If you think you might be at risk, learn as much as you can about the illness before your child is born.
- Share the information with your husband so he's prepared just in case: once a woman is clinically depressed she's not going to have the motivation to do much to help herself.
- My book *Childbirth & Marriage* has an extensive section on PPD. (So few books deal with PPD that I have to be uncouth and plug my own work!)
- Postpartum depression is nothing to be ashamed of: it is a common illness that can be treated.

No support system for the new mother?

- In "the old days" a woman was surrounded by relatives and neighbors when she had a new baby.
- In today's society we are often an airplane ride away from our parents or siblings and have never even met our neighbors!
- A new mom is often cut off from the world outside when she's alone at home with a newborn; isolation is often a cause of depression.
- Once your child is born your closeness to your obstetrician or midwife, which may have been a satisfyingly supportive relationship, usually ends.
- Do you have anyone to turn to for support, advice, and warmth after the baby arrives?

YOU'RE VULNERABLE TO PPD IF . . .

✦ You had PPD after a previous pregnancy.

✦ You had a severe depression at some earlier time.

✦ You've suffered from PMS (premenstrual syndrome).

✦ There is a history of manic-depression in your family; childbirth may trigger depressive illness.

"How can I tell if I'm personally likely to get PPD?"

- You may be carrying a heavy emotional burden without realizing it.
- The chart below identifies stress factors that can lead to postpartum depression.

STRESSES THAT CAN CAUSE POSTPARTUM DEPRESSION

❖ You or your partner are ambivalent about pregnancy

❖ Several previous miscarriages or abortions

❖ History of hormonal problems (early menses; irregular, painful periods; PMS symptoms)

❖ New marriage still in the erotic/romantic stage

❖ Recent move to a new home

❖ First baby

❖ No help available after baby arrives

❖ You're ill, because of pregnancy or not

❖ Death of a parent (mother especially) in childhood or adolescence

❖ Recent death or severe illness of someone close to you

❖ Fears that motherhood will jeopardize your career

❖ You—or your mate—have a new position or increased responsibilities at current job

❖ Partner away from home a great deal

❖ You are accustomed to being out of the house a lot

❖ Marital tension or discord: feeling unloved or unsupported by partner

---

Ways to fight back against PPD

→ Take care of yourself physically. REST when possible; EAT nutritious foods.

→ Get household help: someone to assist with chores *and* to give you a break from the baby.

→ Get out of the house every day so you don't feel trapped or isolated (even if it's only to push the baby buggy around the block).

→ Exercise can give you a lift and an energy boost.

→ Do something nice for yourself every day, preferably away from the baby: take a walk in the park, have a cappuccino while you read the paper, browse in a bookstore, work out in a health club, or stop by a friend's house.

→ Take breaks from the baby just like you would on any job: coffee breaks, lunch break, etc.

→ Use one of the baby's nap times as a chance to pamper yourself with a bubble bath, a nap, a manicure, etc.

→ Crying can be good for you. Try not to resist your sadness: tears can relieve stress and be healing.

YOUR DREAMS

→ During pregnancy your dreams can be more vivid and sometimes disturbing (the father-to-be can have bizarre or puzzling dreams, too).

→ The dream world gives you a chance to explore your feelings about your body, your own mother, your marriage, motherhood, the baby, labor, and delivery.

→ Dreams are stimulated because your subconscious is stirred up by hopes, doubts, and fears. It's a way for you to wrestle with those feelings.

→ Excitement and stress, adjustments and inner conflicts, all surface during sleep.

→ Dreams have a purpose at this time in your life; think of them as messages about yourself, information you can't get any other way.

→ Think of using your dreams to strengthen yourself in getting to know yourself better.

→ You're more impressionable and superstitious right now, so don't get carried away thinking of dreams as being real.

→ Don't panic or be judgmental about fearful feelings. There's nothing weird about you; all this is normal!

Why you're more aware of dreams now

→ At any time of stress or upheaval in a person's life, that person is more aware of dreaming.

→ This is especially true of pregnancy, when there are powerful physical changes along with the mental process.

→ Changes in hormone levels can cause frequent dreaming and/or dreams that seem more vivid with more memorable details.

→ You may remember more of your dreams because of frequent awakening (to go to the bathroom or because of other pregnancy-related discomforts). Frequent waking means better recall of dreams.

PREGNANT DREAMS

THE DREAM IS ABOUT	WHAT IT MAY MEAN
Mistreating the baby	Fear about doing a good parenting job; underlying fear about "doing right" by your child.
Losing the baby	Can represent self-doubt as a good parent; can also be *not* about losing the newborn but losing the baby from your womb, where you've had him all to yourself, safe and sound.
Losing your partner	Inner pressures and external ones like finances can make you feel your relationship is in jeopardy.
Baby dying or malformed	Concern that the baby will not be healthy and perfect; near the end of pregnancy, can be a defense mechanism for fear that something will go wrong with delivery.
Anger toward baby; mental or physical hostility	Nightmares may generally be a way to express resentment toward the unborn child who is going to take over your life, disrupting your privacy and habits.
Baby is a puppy, kitten, or rabbit	Cuddly baby animals often represent the baby; they are stand-ins or symbols in your dreams.
Images of water, tidal waves	May represent amniotic fluid.
Architectural symbols: tunnels, houses, buildings	Some believe these images, along with cars and boats, may represent your own body in your dreams.

PREGNANT NIGHTMARES

✤ Nighttime adventures (even nightmares scary enough to wake you up) are a normal part of pregnancy.

✤ Out-of-control (even monstrous) dreams can be a healthy way to express deep fears.

✤ Dreams with disturbing symbols (snakes, an abnormal baby) or events (a funeral, giving birth to puppies) *do not foretell anything.*

✤ Nightmares can ventilate feelings you cannot express or don't consciously realize you have.

✤ Nightmares are not omens; they have absolutely nothing to do with what is going to happen.

✤ Don't take nightmares literally (no matter how real they seem!) or allow yourself to get superstitious. That's where the saying "It's just a bad dream" comes from; nightmares are something you wake up from and leave to go on to real life.

✤ Don't talk about your dreams to anyone whose emotional reaction might alarm you.

CAN WE TALK?

→ Talk, talk, talk about what you're going through. Pregnancy is a time to indulge yourself and explore your feelings.

→ So much is going on during pregnancy that communicating what you're going through is especially important.

→ When life is confusing or overwhelming, often a good way to figure out what you're feeling is by talking aloud.

→ Unexpressed feelings can get worse if they're bottled up.

→ If no one close to you is pregnant or has small children, it can seem hard to find someone to understand you.

→ Extended family may not be appealing to talk to because old "emotional baggage" can get in the way of really opening up. But you can find out only by giving it a try!

Whose ear to bend

YOUR HUSBAND

Don't hold back. Tell him whatever you're going through; it will bring you closer. Your fears, doubts, and dreams can also free his feelings.

YOUR MOTHER

No one knows you better. Or cares about you more (regardless of thorny times between you in the past). If you've had your differences let this baby be the natural opportunity to bury the hatchet.

SISTER OR CLOSE FRIEND

Even if she hasn't been pregnant, a woman who's close to you is a natural choice for a confidante.

OLDER WOMEN

Your aunt, grandmother, teacher, godmother, and friends of your mother's have the wisdom of personal experience and observation.

CHILDBIRTH EDUCATION TEACHER

Choose your teacher early in pregnancy—then you can call her to talk before classes even begin. A Lamaze teacher has experience dealing with the things that may be affecting you and she can have good advice.

"EARLY BIRD" CLASSES

These are discussion groups designed for prospective parents. It's not easy to find these classes, but they're usually run by the same people in charge of childbirth education. There's some emphasis on practical babycare but the main emphasis is on sharing the impact of pregnancy in your life.

TALK TO YOURSELF!

Get a notebook (or a copy of *The Pregnancy Diary*, which I wrote just for this purpose) and jot down thoughts and feelings. Even if you write only a sentence or two, keeping a journal is a wonderful outlet for feelings, gives you insight into yourself, and will also be a wonderful remembrance of this very special time in your life.

WAYS TO TAKE CARE
OF NUMBER ONE
(P.S. YES! THAT IS YOU!)

It is important to look after yourself: if you're not rested and satisfied you'll have less patience and may feel resentful. Your feelings may come out in the way you deal with the baby, your mate, and/or your career.

Set aside time for yourself and no one else.
You may be amazed at how all-consuming a new baby can be. You'll need to make a point of saving a piece of each day just for yourself.

Set up priorities for yourself.
→ Unless you have help it's impossible to accomplish everything around the house, take care of the baby, and still leave time for yourself.
→ Learn to leave things until "tomorrow." (Or just forget about them until after the baby is toilet-trained!)
→ Don't become a slave to your baby or to housekeeping.

Decide what you will not give up.
It might be an exercise class or playing the piano. Whatever it is that nurtures you should not be lost because of a new baby.

Taking care of number one
→ If you don't take good care of yourself, you can't take good care of your family.
→ You need to feel rested, satisfied with your life, and content within yourself to put out all the energy required of a mother.
→ It's easy to make the mistake of putting your baby and husband first, thinking everything else is more important than your "selfish" needs.
→ *Selfish* is *not* a bad word. Looking after "number one" fulfills you but it also nourishes your whole family.
→ If you don't take care of your own needs, everyone is cheated— unless you feel great you'll have less patience and emotion for your partner and child(ren).

WAYS TO BE GOOD TO YOURSELF

Let others baby you.

When you feel overwhelmed by the demands of motherhood turn to your mate, a friend, or a family member for a dose of "TLC."

Don't expect others to read your mind.

Let people close to you know when you're feeling vulnerable or that you need them in some way. There isn't time anymore for being coy or dropping hints in the hope of being nurtured.

Every day ask "What would be nice for me today?"

It doesn't matter if you can actually carry it out, or even if you always have an answer to the question. What matters is remembering to ask, which is making a point of staying in touch with yourself.

Set aside time for yourself.

Protect a certain piece of each day for yourself. Use the time however you want—paint your toenails, write letters, read, catch up with friends on the phone, nap, daydream to music.

TENSION IN YOUR MARRIAGE

* A couple is often brought closer together by pregnancy, but sometimes the relationship goes through difficult times.
* Going from being individuals who are half of "a couple" to becoming parents who form a family is a big life change.

A new sense of permanence

→ Marriage is already a big commitment; pregnancy can feel like you're putting a permanent seal on that now.
→ No matter how good your relationship is, this new bond may feel a little tight at first.
→ If you feel trapped or cornered, that's normal; it's probably the permanence implied by the expected baby.
→ The impending reality of a baby makes it much harder to imagine just walking away from each other if the going got rough.
  - You'll have the baby's life to consider in everything you do from now on.
  - If either of you is uncomfortable about feeling "tied down" don't take it as a sign there's anything wrong between you.
  - Wrestling with new perceptions of yourself and your union is healthy: facing reality is a sign of maturity.
→ Discussing these feelings with your partner can relieve the pressure.
  - Before sharing your feelings, ask your mate not to view your emotions as a personal rejection.
  - Set the ground rules for being open and honest (or airing your feelings can backfire into a fight!).

The need to depend on someone now

→ You may feel more vulnerable now: let your mate know the feelings you're having.
→ You may find yourself making unusual demands to test your partner's loyalty and devotion.
→ If being independent was important to you before getting pregnant, you may feel stifled by the idea of being *more* closely linked to your husband.
→ Pregnancy heightens a couple's realization of how interdependent they are; you may want to resist the desire to lean on your mate or even pull away.

→ The impulse to withdraw probably won't feel as strong once you realize it's a reaction to feeling too dependent.

Judging each other as future parents

→ You've both fantasized (maybe without realizing it) what kind of Mama or Papa your partner would be.

→ Tension can result from the process of facing the reality of becoming parents; suddenly you see flaws or failings in your partner.

→ Either of you may start criticizing little things about the other person, for no apparent reason.

    • With parenthood around the corner you may not realize you're evaluating "the parent" in each other.

    • Confused, hurt feelings can result if you don't recognize what's going on.

→ Promises you made or beliefs you had before getting pregnant may change now.

    • There's a big difference between theory and reality; don't hold each other to past dinner table declarations about "How It Will Be" when you get pregnant some day.

    • The reality of becoming parents can, for example, alter a man's pre-pregnancy vows that he would change half the diapers or a woman's belief that she would stop working when she became a mother.

    • Give each other the room to grow into more realistic ideas about parenthood—concepts that will probably change time and again after the baby is born!

→ Your partner may have self-doubts about the kind of parent he or she will be.

    • Don't doubt his or her abilities or sincerity because of this self-examination.

    • Be supportive of your mate's willingness to explore feelings and previous assumptions.

MAN'S ADJUSTMENT TO PARENTHOOD

A new father often feels that the baby comes first and gets all the attention. It's important to allow time for yourselves as a couple apart from the baby.

Baby's new father
→ Men are often ignored during their wives' pregnancies: all the attention is focused on the woman.
→ There is often no support system to help prepare an expectant father, but nevertheless he's expected to deal with:
  - His wife's emotional and physical needs
  - New financial burdens
  - His own feelings about becoming a father
→ It's not fair to view a man as a "rock of Gibraltar" now, even if he embraces that role. He shares many of your doubts and fears.

New-age dads
→ The traditional idea of a father meant excluding him from most aspects of pregnancy, birth, and early child care.
→ Nowadays men have the option to become more involved without "risking" their virility or male identity.
→ Expectations have gone in the opposite direction: men are often totally involved now, going on visits to the obstetrician, cutting the umbilical cord, and changing diapers.
→ However, a father-to-be should not feel *obligated* to throw himself into the pregnancy experience. Welcoming him in is not the same as making him feel guilty if he wants less than maximum involvement in the birth or in the baby's development.

Factors That Influence a Father's Adjustment

Preparation for parenting	Men feel inadequate because they don't know how to feed, bathe, or diaper a baby. Attending infant-care demonstrations at a hospital or through the American Red Cross can prevent a man from feeling shut out of his baby's early months.
Agreement about roles	Men tend to adopt either the Breadwinner role or the Equal Parent role. Either is fine as long as both partners feel comfortable.
Support from his workplace	A man should talk to his employers before the baby is born to get some flexibility with his hours in the early months after birth.
Support from your families	The support of one's family or extended family can be a great comfort. Feeling that you aren't all alone out there means a lot.

A New Dad's Fears

Finances

❖ Money issues like insurance and budgeting are often considered the man's domain.

❖ A man can focus too much on finances.

❖ Concentrating on money issues can be a way to avoid deeper worries, like being a competent father.

❖ A father-to-be can share his wife's doubts about being able to care properly for the baby—but express the fear by concentrating on finances.

❖ This is similar to a woman who has food cravings to express her need for attention.

Loss of independence

✤ A woman can have more emotional and physical needs during pregnancy because of her changing identity.

✤ A man can be frightened by his wife's leaning more heavily on him now.

✤ A man's sense of freedom can be threatened by the increased feelings of being needed.

✤ He may also be unsure of whether he will be able to give his wife the emotional support she needs.

✤ In the last trimester the man's anxiety about being "leaned on" may intensify; the baby's room is being assembled and a woman may be less able to do normal tasks around the house.

Sex

✤ Often a man has less sex drive when his wife is pregnant.

✤ Some reasons for this drop in sexual desire:
  • Fear of harming the fetus (even with medical reassurance that sex can't hurt the baby).
  • Discomfort with changes in the woman's body (what she looks like outside and feels like inside) can make a man pull away.
  • The idea of "mother" doesn't fit with his image of a sexual partner.
  • If the woman has increased sex drive, more lubrication, or a greater ability to be orgasmic the man can feel overwhelmed, inadequate to satisfy her.

✤ Consider alternatives to intercourse:
  • Oral or manual sex might seem less threatening.
  • Substitutes for penetration can lower inhibitions (and sometimes lead to intercourse).
  • Any form of sexual activity brings you closer (if both partners are comfortable with it, obviously).

✤ Talk about what's going on for you sexually; encourage your partner to express his reactions.
  • Discussing sex can be difficult for some people.
  • Open communication about your changing needs and feelings is as intimate as sex itself.
  • Sharing feelings, even negative ones, can bring you closer together.
  • Talking freely about what you're going through can make problems seem less intense.

Envy and jealousy
→ A man may not be aware that he's feeling jealous of his pregnant wife.
→ Envy can affect a man in disguised ways.
→ A man can have an unconscious longing to experience pregnancy and birth.
  ⋙ This can lead to bursts of creativity or a stronger drive to accomplish.
  ⋙ These can be ways to sublimate the desire to be pregnant.
→ A woman's new closeness to her mother (or other female friend or relative) can make a man feel jealous.
→ He may feel shut out, fearful his wife doesn't trust him as much as before.
→ If a man feels displaced he needs reassurance.
→ He needs to realize that his wife's closeness to someone else does not jeopardize her attachment to him.

Motherly, nurturant feelings
→ Many men feel more protective and gentle when their wives are pregnant.
→ A man is learning to "mother" his wife when he looks after her in new ways and does additional tasks.
→ If her parents are deceased or live far away, the man may become the main "mothering figure" for his wife.
→ Identifying with a feminine part of themselves can be frightening to some men:
  ⋙ Pregnancy triggers a man's ability to be nurturant.
  ⋙ This identification can be so worrisome that it causes impotence for some men.
  ⋙ Others may counteract this fear by throwing themselves into work or supermasculine (macho) endeavors.
→ Instead of being more nurturing a man may take on extra chores or ready the house for the baby's arrival.

Practice for parenting
→ Being nurturant with his wife is a way to be more involved with the pregnancy and to practice being a father.
→ By supporting his mate through pregnancy and delivery a man is also preparing himself for fatherhood.
→ By getting in touch with his motherliness a man can respond better to his baby.

→ A man can get a lot of pleasure from nurturing if the woman (and later the baby) are receptive to him.

The paternal role

→ A man has to prepare himself for his new role.

→ He may be worried about playing this new part.

→ He'll probably be more relaxed about developing as a father if his relationship with his own father has been good.

→ If his relationship with his father was negative, a man may distrust his own abilities to be a parent.

→ Talking about what he liked and disliked in his relationship with his father will help him form an image in his own mind of what a good father should be.

→ Being there for his baby's birth can arouse a man's paternal feelings and create a bond that encourages him to participate in taking care of the baby later.

Pulling away

→ A man's disinterest in pregnancy and childbirth is not a sign of a problem in your relationship; he may feel overwhelmed.

    ❧ Don't treat his withdrawal as an attack on you or the baby.

    ❧ Don't get hurt or disappointed, which will just add guilt to the confusion of his feelings.

    ❧ Taking a superior attitude will only reinforce his feeling of inadequacy and drive him further away.

→ Men often feel excluded and uninformed about childbearing.

    ❧ Offer him this book or other information so he feels more on top of what's going on inside you.

    ❧ Be compassionate. What would you feel like if *you* were the one on the outside, not the center of the experience?

→ A man may not want to participate in labor and delivery.

    ❧ Ask him to go to one childbirth class with you and see if he feels any better.

    ❧ Don't force or wheedle him into a decision against his will.

    ❧ Your enthusiasm about how great it's going to be, or criticism of him for not wanting to be there, will turn him off even more.

    ❧ Respect his feelings (even if you don't like them!) and choose someone else to be your coach.

    ❧ By giving him room and not being judgmental you allow your partner to change his mind gracefully.

- Remember, many wonderful fathers have not been present for their babies' births. Being at his child's birth does not automatically mean a man will be a better father.
→ Various fears may be causing a man to pull away.
    - **Fear of the unknown:** The more he can learn about the childbearing experience, the less he'll feel intimidated.
    - **Fear of hospitals:** Many people are frightened by hospitals because of a personal bad experience or because they represent sickness and death. Take the official tour, maybe more than once; getting familiar with the place can alleviate fears.
    - **Fear of inadequacy:** If a man is squeamish he may be afraid he won't handle himself well during the messy parts of childbirth (have him talk to other new fathers who "survived"). Or he may worry about being able to meet his wife's emotional needs during the intensity of labor (reassure him that just his being there will make you feel better).
    - **Overcoming fears** can be as simple as reassurance from you, or hearing other people's childbirth experiences.

Running away

→ Some men feel so overwhelmed by the external and emotional demands of impending parenthood that they run away.
→ This is more than withdrawing; it is a literal or figurative attempt to put distance between themselves and you.
→ These men find excuses: longer working hours, sports events they "must" participate in, business trips, etc.
→ Beware the way you react to feeling ignored and/or abandoned.
    - A pregnant woman's reaction to her absentee husband can set a vicious cycle in motion.
    - You're likely to drive him further away if you insist that he spend more time with you, or if you become emotionally dramatic to get his attention.
    - If you make demands you're increasing the pressure he's already trying to escape. He'll feel more suffocated or inadequate or angry.
→ A man who is running is in danger of having an affair.
    - Starting an affair is a way to prove his independence to himself.
    - An affair is also a way to assert his denial of what is happening at home and how his life is about to change.

- Professional counseling is the most effective way for a man on the run to stop and understand what's "chasing" him.

Becoming a workaholic

→ Work can take on a new importance for a man who's an expectant parent.

→ A man may throw himself into work for many reasons:
- an unconscious desire to procreate, to give birth himself.
- an increased awareness of his duties as a provider and the need to bring in more money now.
- a way to avoid facing his doubts about becoming a father.

→ Work is an area where he feels competent and safe, which he may not feel about pregnancy and childbirth.

→ Throwing himself into work may help a man figure things out.
- Each man has to do the best he can to deal with unfamiliar feelings.
- Work is one area where a man can express complicated feelings he doesn't understand.
- Don't view his intensity about work as necessarily bad; it may be part of his process of growth and learning.

→ Don't view his increased hours of work as a rejection of you.
- Don't get hung up on his long hours working because once the baby is born *your* time will be limited.
- Diminished time together is going to be part of your new life with a baby.

→ Begin to view your time together for its quality, not its quantity. Make an effort for that time to be relaxing, interesting, and pleasurable.

10.
The Big Day

Giving Birth

It's here! The moment you've been waiting for
... planning for ... dreading a little ... eager to
experience! The more you know ahead of time
about the process of labor and delivery, the
more you can participate in this tremendous
moment when it arrives.

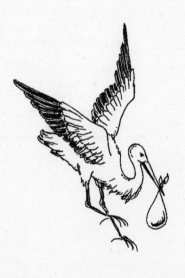

SIGNS OF PRELABOR

Lightening (also called "engagement")	Takes place two to three weeks before labor. The baby's presenting part (usually the head) is "engaged" in the pelvis. In a woman who has already had a baby, lightening may not occur until early in labor. Breathing may be easier after engagement. You may need to urinate more frequently because of increased pressure on your bladder.
Braxton-Hicks contractions	These are "practice" contractions that are more common during first pregnancies. The uterus is flexing its muscles to prepare for labor.
Increased vaginal mucus	"Bloody show," which is the rupture of the mucus plug blocking the cervix, is usually a sign of early labor, although it can occur as much as twelve days before labor begins.
Weight loss	A weight loss of two to three pounds often occurs three to four days before the onset of labor.
Excess energy	Some women experience a rush of energy, which motivates them to do extra chores. *Resist* this urge and conserve the energy for labor.

SIGNS OF FALSE LABOR

Contractions may subside
Walking and standing during true labor causes contractions to worsen.

During false labor they may subside.

The intensity diminishes
In false labor, contractions reach a plateau and the intensity diminishes.

In true labor they get stronger and longer.

Call your doctor
They can often tell from your voice during a contraction whether it's the real thing.

A good rule of thumb
If you need to use breathing techniques during a contraction, you're probably in labor.

Get medical reassurance
If you're concerned, go to the hospital so they can check if your cervix is opening. Do not be embarrassed if you are told it is not true labor.

WHAT TO PACK IN YOUR HOSPITAL BAG

+ Two nightgowns (front opening, if you're breast-feeding) and a robe and slippers for walking around.
+ Two nursing bras.
+ Baby clothes—nightgown or stretch suit; receiving blanket.
+ Sanitary pads and belt—if you don't want to pay the hospital for each one they issue.
+ Camera—ask the hospital beforehand if you need permission forms.
+ Heavy socks—it can be cold in the delivery room.

WHEN TO CALL THE DOCTOR

✤ If during the space of an hour the contractions are fifteen minutes apart and last for one minute.

✤ If contractions don't go away when you move around.

✤ Don't rush to the hospital: the first stage of labor lasts an average of eight and a half hours with a first baby.

✤ When to leave for the hospital: with a first baby, when the contractions are about a minute long; otherwise, when the first level of breathing is no longer adequate.

✤ Be familiar with the hospital route and know which entrance you need to use.

STAGES OF LABOR:
WHAT'S HAPPENING,
HOW TO COPE

FIRST-STAGE LABOR: DILATION

* In the first stage of labor your cervix is dilated by the uterine contractions.
* Dilation is the opening of the cervix so that the baby can pass through into the birth canal.
* Dilation is measured in centimeters; the cervix is completely open at ten centimeters.
* When the cervix is fully dilated the first stage of labor is complete.

Signs of first-stage labor

→ Your membranes may rupture
  ❧ Membranes usually rupture late in first-stage labor.
  ❧ It does not hurt; you will feel only a warm flow of water.
→ Pink show (also called "bloody show")
  The blood-tinged mucus plug that was blocking the cervix breaks loose before labor.
→ Length of contractions
  ❧ Contractions are timed from the *beginning* of one contraction to the *beginning* of the next.
  ❧ In early labor they are thirty to sixty seconds long with five to twenty minutes between contractions.
  ❧ This is the stage of labor that lasts an average of eight and a half hours for first babies.
→ Late first-stage (or active-phase) labor
  ❧ In the *active phase* of labor the cervix opens from four to seven centimeters.
  ❧ The contractions are forty-five to seventy-five seconds long and two to four minutes apart.
  ❧ After about five centimeters of dilation your prepared breathing techniques usually become necessary to maintain comfort.

Transition

→ The time before you are fully dilated is known as "transition": from the end of first-stage labor to the beginning of the second stage, when you'll be pushing the baby out.

→ Transition occurs when you are seven to eight centimeters dilated. It may last no more than ten to thirty contractions.

→ This is the hardest part of labor but it is also the shortest: the *average* length of transition with a first baby is one and a half hours, but it usually lasts no more than thirty to sixty minutes.

→ You'll need extra encouragement from your partner during this stage of labor, which can be the most emotionally demanding time.

→ Oxygen is being concentrated in the uterus rather than the brain, which means there's more need for your coach to alert you that a contraction is coming and for breathing coaching during the contractions.

→ It's helpful to look for the signs of transition, which means you'll be ready to push soon. There are many signs, of which a woman may have many or only a few.

SIGNS OF TRANSITION

✤ Discouragement   "I can't go on."

✤ Shaking, shivering   Don't resist or be frightened by it.

✤ Irritability   "Don't touch me, get away."

✤ Nausea   Don't resist vomiting: you'll feel better afterward.

✤ Restlessness

✤ Excitement

✤ Disorientation

✤ Anxiety for your safety and the baby's

✤ Dizziness

✤ Prickly skin (especially on fingers)

✤ Sleepiness between contractions

→ Transition is the emotional booby trap of labor: many women lose faith in their own abilities and prepared childbirth techniques and turn to medications.

→ Transition is the ultimate test of how well a woman and her coach are working together. Give her a pep talk now:

  ❧ EXPLAIN THAT HER LOSS OF FAITH is normal during transition, which is the roughest part but will be over soon.

  ❧ TELL HER HOW WELL SHE HAS DONE UNTIL NOW and that transition means first-stage labor is almost over and soon she'll be pushing out her baby.

  ❧ REMIND HER IT WILL ONLY BE A LITTLE LONGER and this increased discomfort is only temporary.

  ❧ EXPLAIN THAT CONTRACTIONS ARE ERRATIC during transition because they come close together and may have 3 or 4 peaks and be hard to manage—but she shouldn't lose faith!

  ❧ TELL HER HOW IMPORTANT CONCENTRATION is now: if she isn't ready for a contraction she may panic and doubt she can go on with her techniques for breathing and relaxation.

  ❧ HELP HER FOCUS on the current so that she doesn't lose control because she's thinking about a previous contraction or worrying about what's coming up.

→ The end of transition is often marked by a catch in your labor breathing—it may be a sound like a hiccup. This means the bearing-down reflex is beginning to be established and you'll have the urge to push soon.

Backache

→ Backache during labor is experienced by a majority of women; it is severe for only a few.

→ Most women have backache during transition.

→ There are three techniques for relieving backache:

  ❧ **Counterpressure** involves making a fist and putting it under your back where the pressure is worst, pressing down during contractions.

  ❧ **A position change** that gets the baby off your spine will relieve or reduce pressure.

  ❧ **Application of heat,** either during or between contractions, helps some women.

Examination during labor

→ Examinations during labor are done periodically to check for dilation and the baby's position.

→ Ask how you are progressing after each exam.

→ If contractions are getting longer and stronger and you haven't been checked for a while *ask for an examination.*

→ Your coach may be asked to leave during an exam, presumably for reasons of "modesty."

→ Explain that you need your coach during contractions and you'd appreciate not being separated from him.

Dilation of the cervix in centimeters

This is a life-size diagram of how much your cervix opens.

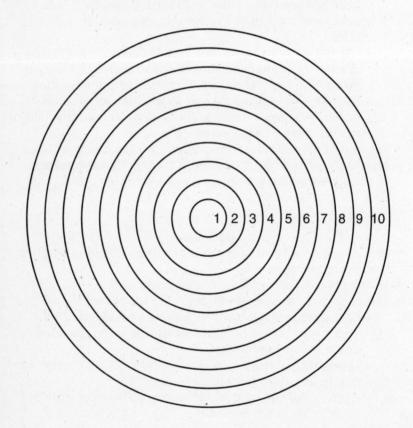

SECOND-STAGE LABOR: PUSHING TO BIRTH

* The second stage of labor lasts from complete dilation of your cervix until the baby is born.
* This is the pushing stage of the labor, usually lasting one to three hours for a first baby
* In subsequent deliveries, pushing usually lasts 30 to 60 minutes.

The urge to push
→ Many women feel an overwhelming urge to push.
→ Do not push until you have been examined to make sure you are fully dilated.
→ You may have to use a "pant" or "blow" breathing technique to avoid pushing until you're told it is safe.

Contractions
→ They are usually four to five minutes apart.
→ Each contraction lasts about a minute.
→ It is during the contraction that you push.
→ Begin your pushing effort with the peak intensity of each contraction.

Relaxation of anal area
→ Make a conscious effort to relax this part of your body when pushing to get the maximum benefit from your efforts.
→ Don't worry about bowel movements: the attendants have seen it all before!

Positions for pushing
→ The hospital usually encourages lying on the back or a semi-sitting position.
→ If you have tried other positions at home ahead of time and would prefer kneeling, squatting, being on hands and knees, or lying on your side, tell the attendant.

After two hours of pushing
→ Most doctors intervene after two hours of pushing.
→ You may be too exhausted to continue and it is hard for the baby to stay in the birth canal that long.
→ In this case a forceps delivery is usual.

Giving birth in the labor room
→ This is an option to discuss with your doctor ahead of time.
→ One benefit is being spared the rushed transfer to the delivery room.
→ Also you save money—the birth itself can cost half as much.
→ However, if there is any indication that your baby is in distress it is preferable to move to a delivery room.

The transfer to the delivery table
→ The labor bed is pushed alongside the delivery table and you have to shift sideways.
→ The move is clumsy; you may lose your pushing rhythm.
→ Try to relax.
→ It is best not to make the move during a contraction.

Face masks
→ Everyone in the delivery room will wear one except you.
→ This is for the baby's protection.

Stirrups
→ Stirrups are used in most delivery rooms to support your legs.
→ You can ask to have them adjusted lower so your legs are more comfortable.

Mirror
→ A mirror above the delivery table allows you to watch the baby coming out.
→ Push with open eyes: many women squeeze their eyes shut when they are pushing hard and miss the sight of their baby emerging.

The birth itself
→ With each contraction more and more of the head shows, receding back into the birth canal between contractions.
→ Don't get discouraged; you push the baby down "two steps" and she slides back one.
→ Once the head is out the baby will turn to her side, putting the shoulders in a position to be born easily.

THIRD-STAGE LABOR: PLACENTA

The third stage of labor is the delivery of the placenta.

Doctors are often impatient
→ They may wish to get the placenta to expel in a few minutes, even though it normally takes twenty to thirty minutes.
→ If a doctor says that he has to perform a manual removal after only ten minutes without a medical reason, ask him to wait.
→ Manual removal can cause hemorrhage.

If the placenta doesn't detach spontaneously
→ The doctor and nurse will push on your abdomen.
→ In a case like this the doctor should explain that the placenta is not detaching and that he has to go in and get it.
→ This is different from a doctor who rushes in to perform a manual removal because he is impatient.
→ This can be uncomfortable; you may need to use the breathing techniques you used during first-stage labor.

Examination of the placenta
→ The placenta is examined to make sure it is complete and none was left behind.
→ If any piece of placenta is left in your uterus it can cause hemorrhage later on.

Shaking after birth
→ This is normal and can sometimes be quite strong.
→ The big drop in hormones is probably the reason.
→ Don't be frightened; ask for a blanket and try to relax.

The recovery room
→ You will be sent to the recovery room for one to three hours after delivery.
→ A nurse will check your pulse and blood pressure and knead your uterus to make sure it remains firm.

Hunger
→ You may be ravenous after the birth of your baby.
→ The hospital may serve food only at designated mealtimes.
→ If you're starving you might have to persuade a relative to make a food run for you.

MEDICATIONS USED FOR LABOR AND DELIVERY

Think before you ask for medication

→ The American Academy of Pediatrics recommends the least possible medication during childbirth.

→ All drugs except epidural anesthesia reach your baby.

→ However, an epidural affects your labor, and therefore can affect your baby.

→ Consider the "price tag" of drugs before you take any.

→ Fetal monitors show patterns of oxygen deprivation to the babies of women taking Demerol, which is a pain medication, and oxytocin, a synthetic hormone to speed up contractions.

→ You have the legal right to refuse all medication.

→ Try to wait fifteen minutes to half an hour after you think you want drugs before taking them.

There are times when medication is helpful.

→ The foremost reason for accepting drugs is if you become very tense and cannot relax.

→ Tension can slow down labor, which can cause fetal distress.

→ There is a growing belief among doctors that prolonged pain in the mother can affect the baby as well.

→ Advanced technology means that much more is known today about how drugs interact with the baby.

→ Doctors today are giving smaller doses of medications.

There are three types of medications used for childbirth.

→ Analgesic is used for pain relief.

→ Oxytocics are used to induce labor or speed it up.

→ Anesthetics are used locally to numb that area.

MEDICATION USED DURING LABOR

Analgesics
(to relieve pain)

**Tranquilizers
(Miltown, Vistaril, Phenergan, Largon, Sparine)**

✤ Reduce anxiety

✤ Good for long labors if tension mounts

✤ May have little effect on fetus

✤ Excess can cause loss of control over contractions

✤ NOTE: Valium should not be given because of the length of time it remains in the newborn's body.

**Barbiturates
(Seconal, Nembutal)**

✤ Sedates and produces sleep

✤ Effects on the newborn last up to a week after birth

**Narcotics
(Demerol, Phentinyl, Dolophine)**

✤ Relieve pain, sedate, relieve anxiety

✤ Negative effect on the newborn's respiration

**Amnesics
(scopolamine)**

✤ Used in combination with pain-relieving drugs

✤ Hallucinogenic

✤ Drawbacks outweigh any advantages

✤ Causes violent, odd behavior

**Inhalation analgesia
(nitrous oxide, Penthrane, Trilene)**

✤ Inhaled during peak of contraction

✤ Self-administered

✤ Have to learn to time self-administration so maximum effect coincides with peak of contraction

Oxytocics
(to induce or speed up labor)

Pitocin
- ✤ The most commonly used oxytocic
- ✤ Often given through the IV. The doctor cannot easily control the dosage when administered this way.
- ✤ The alternate method is through your vein via infusion pump. With this method the doctor can increase or decrease the dosage instantly depending on how your body reacts.

Ergotrate
- ✤ Oxytocic given in pill form after delivery to contract your uterus
- ✤ If you are breast-feeding, the hormones that will contract the uterus are naturally excreted

Anesthesia

General anesthesia
- ✤ Seldom used in normal births
- ✤ Inhaled to produce unconsciousness
- ✤ Forceps necessary
- ✤ Side effects include grogginess and amnesia

All other anesthesia is regional (local)

Caudal
- ✤ Administered in your lower back after six centimeters' dilation
- ✤ You are turned on your side while a thin tube is inserted and taped in place
- ✤ Blocks sensation but you can usually still move
- ✤ Removes the urge to bear down but trained women can still push
- ✤ Passes quickly to baby and can cause a drop in maternal blood pressure, which can affect baby's oxygen supply
- ✤ Forceps often required
- ✤ Risk of puncturing rectum or baby's head

Epidural	✛ Administered after six centimeters' dilation in a procedure similar to caudal
	✛ Does not cross placenta
	✛ Thought to be the safest drug with minimal side effects
	✛ You can feel pressure but not pain, yet you lose the urge to push
	✛ 75 percent of epidural deliveries use forceps
	✛ 25 percent of babies show dramatic slow-down in heart rate when given in early labor
	✛ Epidural necessitates the following:
	• IV hydrating solution
	• Blood pressure taken every fifteen to thirty minutes
	• Fetal monitoring—to monitor baby's reaction and tolerance to it
Spinal	✛ Injected into spinal fluid at eight centimeters or after full dilation (i.e. no relief of first-stage labor)
	✛ Necessary to lie flat on your back for four to eight hours after delivery
	✛ Used when mother is too tired to push.
	✛ Does not cross placenta
	✛ Relaxes tense perineal area for forceps delivery
	✛ Slows labor as contractions weaken
	✛ Blood pressure drops, reducing oxygen to baby
	✛ Forceps often necessary
Saddle block	✛ Injected into spinal fluid lower than a spinal
	✛ Given close to delivery
	✛ Deadens area you would touch with a saddle
	✛ Less drug required than for a spinal
	✛ Drug does not cross placenta
	✛ Can lower mother's blood pressure
	✛ Can cause spinal headache, even if you lie on your back for twenty minutes afterward

Paracervical block	✜ Administered on side of cervix—active labor must be under way but still some cervix remaining
	✜ Stops pain from uterus and cervix
	✜ Good for cervix not dilating well
	✜ Lasts about one hour but crosses placenta in about three minutes
	✜ Fetal heart rate can slow; can be accidentally injected into fetus
Pudendal block	✜ Injected into pudendal nerve in vagina or into buttocks
	✜ Numbs vagina and perineum (area between vagina and anus)
	✜ Urge to push usually lost but you can still push when told
	✜ Transfers to baby in fifteen minutes
Local infiltration for episiotomy	✜ Xylocaine or procaine injected into perineum
	✜ "Local" only in terms of where it's given
	✜ Reaches entire system instantly

PSYCHOLOGICAL ASPECTS
OF LABOR

* The way you feel and *think* before you go into labor (and while you're in it) influences the physical progress.
* The more informed you are about what to expect, the less anxiety you'll have during birth.
* The more relaxed you are the easier the birth; for this reason having people around you for support is so important.
* Never be left alone when you're in labor.
* However you get through labor is an accomplishment, with or without medication, with a cesarean or not.

NOTES FOR THE COACH

Early labor

→ Encourage her to sleep or conserve energy.
→ Suggest a warm, relaxing bath if her membranes have not broken and you are still at home.
→ Encourage her to drink, unless she is feeling sick. Natural fruit juice is good.
→ When contractions begin, time them. Note the interval between contractions and how long they last.
→ Contractions are timed from the beginning of one contraction to the beginning of the next.
→ Also note if she has any "bloody show."
→ Coaching her through her contractions is your primary task.
→ Make sure each breath is complete, with an emphasis on exhalation, not inhalation.
→ Breathe with her when the going gets rough, establishing eye contact.
→ Remind her to empty her bladder every hour; a full bladder can cause pain during contractions.

Transition

→ Transition is the hardest part of labor.

→ Try to get her to relax.

→ Wipe her face with a cool cloth if she seems warm.

→ If she feels sick get a basin; encourage her to vomit.

→ If her legs are trembling put socks on her, cover her with blankets, and hold her legs firmly.

→ If she grunts or makes pushing movements during a contraction notify the nurse.

→ These are signs that she wants to push; she will need to be examined to insure that her cervix is fully dilated before pushing is safe.

→ She may be cranky and touchy; don't take it personally.

The delivery

→ Teamwork during the delivery phase is now focused between the woman and her doctor.

→ Your role now becomes more one of an observer, although you can still be involved.

→ Change into sterile clothing *before* the transfer to the delivery room so you don't miss anything.

→ Remind her to relax her pelvic floor during pushing.

→ She should take two or three deep breaths and push her hardest at the peak of the contractions.

→ Remind her to look in the mirror at the baby coming out.

→ If asked to leave the delivery room, do so without question (in a medical emergency you will be in the way).

LABOR POSITIONS

Supine position
(lying flat on your back)

- This is the most popular position used in U.S. hospitals.
- There are drawbacks to this position:
    - The normal intensity of contractions is decreased.
    - It inhibits your efforts to push the baby out because gravity is not working in your favor.
    - It increases the need for an episiotomy because it stretches the perineal tissue.
- You might want to try a sitting, semi-sitting, or side-lying position for at least part of your labor.

Dorsal position

- This involves lying on your back with the soles of your feet flat on the delivery table.
- Contraction intensity and effective pushing are not affected as much as in the supine position.
- This position permits your spine to curve so you are working with gravity in pushing the baby out.

Side-lying position

- This takes the weight of your uterus off the main blood supply to the baby.
- It reduces tension on the perineum.
- In the delivery room your right leg can be placed in the stirrup, making this position less tiring.
- The problem with this position is you might have difficulty seeing the mirror to observe the baby coming out.

Semi-sitting position

- Your upper body is propped at a 45-degree angle with your knees flexed and your feet flat on the table.
- Some delivery tables can be adjusted to support your back; otherwise use pillows.
- In this position the force of gravity helps in the descent of the baby.

Hands-and-knees position

- This position takes the weight of the uterus off your back.
- This position can be dangerous for delivery because the baby emerges face up: the amniotic fluid that remains in the uterus can flood over his body and into his mouth and nose.

Birthing chair

- This chair was specially designed for labor and delivery; it may be available in some hospitals.
- Some women like sitting up for delivery.
- Doctors usually dislike the chair because of the difficulty in doing episiotomy repair.

TRANSITION

* This is the time in labor before you are fully dilated.
* It is the transition from the end of first-stage labor to the time when you will be pushing out your baby.
* Transition is the hardest part of labor, but it is also the shortest.
* It occurs when you are seven to eight centimeters dilated and may last only ten to thirty contractions.
* Contractions are erratic, lasting anywhere from 50 to 120 seconds, with three or four peaks.
* They are from 30 seconds to 3 minutes apart.

Signs of transition

- There are many signs of transition. A woman may have a few or many of them:
  - Discouragement ("I can't go on")
  - Shaking, shivering (this is normal and should not be resisted)
  - Nausea (to the point of vomiting)
  - Dizziness or sleepiness between contractions
  - Prickly skin (especially on the fingers)
  - Backache (many women have continuous backache, making relaxation more difficult)

End of transition

- The end of transition is often marked by a catch in your labor breathing.
- This means that you'll have the urge to push soon.
- At this point you should be propped up if you aren't already.
- This allows gravity to help you to move the baby down and out.

EPISIOTOMY

- An episiotomy is an incision made in the perineum, the area between your vagina and anus.
- In American hospitals almost every woman giving birth gets an episiotomy. In hospitals in other countries the rate is around 10 percent.
- Opponents of routine episiotomy claim that positioning women for delivery in a supine position, in stirrups, and in a rush *creates* this need to cut the perineum.
- The technique of massaging the perineum with warm compresses and oil is used by midwives worldwide to help stretch the perineum and reduce tearing of the vagina. Few American doctors or nurses practice this.
- The healing period for episiotomies is uncomfortable; the stitches usually cause itching and pain.

VALID REASONS FOR EPISIOTOMY

- ✤ The perineal tissue hasn't had enough time to stretch gradually, even with the help of massage.
- ✤ The baby's head is too large for the opening.
- ✤ The woman's pushing isn't in perfect control and coordination with the person catching the baby (she is not able to stop pushing when necessary or able to be smooth and gradual when she does push).
- ✤ A speedy delivery is necessary—that is, there are signs of fetal distress.
- ✤ A tear seems imminent (a tear is more difficult to repair than an incision).

CUTTING THE CORD

- Clamping and cutting the umbilical cord are done forty-five seconds to one minute after the birth of the baby.
- The cord is clamped in two places and cut between the clamps.
- Many fathers enjoy cutting the cord; discuss this with your doctor ahead of time.
- There is some debate about whether to cut the cord right away or the more recent practice of "late cord clamping."
- Late cord clamping is believed to allow an increased blood supply to the newborn.

THE NEWBORN

- The newborn is wiped off immediately to prevent cold stress.
- Suctioning with a rubber bulb is usually done when the baby's head is born, even before the body is fully out.
- The baby's mouth and nose are filled with mucus and amniotic fluid; when they are cleared out the baby can breathe easier.
- Antibiotic ointment is applied to the baby's eyes to guard against eye infection.
- Vitamin K is routinely given by injection to newborns because they are deficient in intestinal flora-bacteria. (Breast-fed babies will receive intestinal flora-bacteria; if you do not like the idea of the vitamin K shot, discuss this with your pediatrician ahead of time.)
- A band will be put on your baby with your name and the doctor's name.

Apgar rating
- Apgar rating of the baby is done at one minute after birth and again at five minutes.
- This is a two-point test that rates five aspects of the newborn; heart rate, respiratory effort (a "cry"), muscle tone, reflex irritability, and color.

- The five-minute score gives a more accurate resul: a low score at five minutes is much more serious than the same score at one minute.
- The Apgar rating is only *one* indicator of the baby's well-being. Many birth attendants have a broader checklist by which they evaluate a newborn.

BONDING TO THE BABY

What does the term "bonding" actually mean?

- In the first hour of life the baby is alert and quiet. This time is most rewarding for skin-to-skin and eye-to-eye contact.
- Bonding should be a private session with a minimum of interruptions.
- A newborn with drugs in his system from labor and/or delivery will not be as responsive.
- Studies have shown that a newborn will adapt more easily when she is soothed, held, and given the opportunity to suck at will.
- Father-baby contact is important because a man may need more exposure to the infant to feel as close as the mother.

EXERCISE PROGRAMS
FOR INFANTS

Is this just a fad, or something useful?

→ Structured exercise classes for babies have become increasingly popular in America.
  - Most programs involve massage and passive exercise.
→ The American Academy of Pediatrics recommends *against* these programs.
  - Many pediatricians oppose putting pressure on parents to accelerate a child's normal development.
  - Doctors fear that "the possibility exists that adults may inadvertently exceed the infant's limitations."
→ Some programs involve purchasing equipment and instructional materials.
  - The promoters often claim this will enhance the baby's "quiet alert" states and enhance learning.
  - There are claims of improving an infant's physical abilities or intelligence.
→ Most pediatricians see these classes as part of the Super Baby Syndrome.
  - Health-care professionals believe it's important for a baby to have a stimulating, loving environment.
  - However, no special equipment or skills are necessary.
→ Allow your child to blossom naturally at her own pace....You'll both be a lot happier!

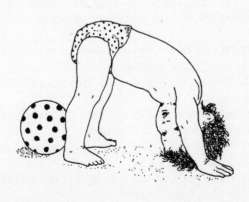

DANGERS TO BABIES
AND SMALL CHILDREN

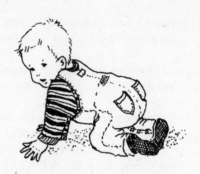

* This section is a collection of miscellaneous dangers to babies and children.
* New parents are rarely alerted to these hazards, so they're included here as a precaution.

Swimming lessons

→ Swim classes for babies only a few months old present dangers that parents are not told.
  - "Forced infant submersion" is the technique often used by instructors to get the baby's face wet.
  - Children have been permanently harmed or have died from water intoxication, which happens when the child takes in too much water.
  - Even if the child does not seem affected at the time of the swimming lesson, this reaction can occur hours or days later.
  - The infant can have convulsions or seizures, go into shock, or even become comatose.
→ The most dangerous classes are the ones for children under the age of three.
  - The biggest risk is classes that claim to "waterproof" or "drownproof" infants and toddlers.
  - Children three and under are at the age most vulnerable to drowning.
  - Children that age can learn to propel themselves in the water but don't understand water safety.

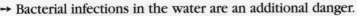

→ Bacterial infections in the water are an additional danger.
  ‌• Kiddie swim classes are held in water used by other children who may be ill.
  ‌• Your child can get an ear infection, sinus condition, and/or bacteria in his lungs.
  ‌• Experts recommend that parents avoid submerging any child until she has developed immunities to bacteria.
→ Experts also suggest that there is substantial physical and mental growth needed before a child attempts swimming.

Waterbeds
→ Waterbeds are dangerous for babies less than two years old.
→ Infants this age cannot turn over on a waterbed.
  ‌• They run the risk of smothering.
  ‌• It takes a tragically short time for an infant to suffocate.
→ Do not leave a young child of any age unattended on a waterbed.
  ‌• If your child is under two do not even turn your back on her.
  ‌• Better yet, just keep your child(ren) off a waterbed while the are little.

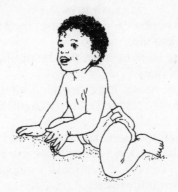

Bath support rings
→ These gadgets can be lethal for babies.
→ Support rings are devices to use in your bathtub for the baby.
→ The rings are usually constructed with three to four legs with suction cups.
→ The suction cups can suddenly release from the bottom of the tub, allowing the device to tip over into the water with a baby in it.

→ A baby can also slip between the legs of the device and get trapped in the water underneath the ring.

→ A baby can drown in the time it takes you to go get a towel.

→ THE MANUFACTURER'S WARNING IS DEADLY SERIOUS: An adult should be present constantly when a baby is in the bath ring.

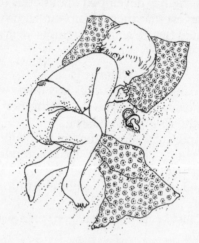

Crib toys

→ Crib toys consist of objects that are stretched across the crib or that dangle from mobiles.

→ Some crib toys are so dangerous that babies have hung themselves on these devices.

→ A tragic number of babies have strangled, suffered brain damage, or been narrowly rescued from strangulation because of these playthings.

    ↞ These contraptions look cute but beware: some are more dangerous than others ... *but none are safe!*

    ↞ These things can cause strangulation once a baby is old enough to reach for them.

    ↞ Most of the victims are over five months old.

    ↞ A dire hazard exists with any and all crib toys, particularly once the baby is older than five months.

→ ***Remove all crib toys strung across the crib or playpen.***

    ↞ Do this when your child is beginning to push up on hands and knees or once the child reaches five months— whichever occurs first.

11.
Cesarean Birth

One out of every ten women will have a
cesarean birth. Many women do not know they
are going to have a cesarean until partway
through labor. Knowing what to expect can
make the procedure less frightening or
discouraging.

INCREASE IN THE CESAREAN RATE

Why are there so many more cesarean sections?

* A cesarean has become so safe that it is considered more risk-free than many complications of vaginal labor and delivery.
* Ultrasound and fetal monitors can predict which babies will be at risk from vaginal delivery, or which babies are in distress once labor has begun.
* Many doctors are afraid of malpractice suits. Parents have backed doctors into a corner. People expect a "perfect" baby and blame the doctor for any errors of nature.
* Doing a C-section gives the doctor more control over the outcome of the birth.

Indications for a cesarean

There are several categories of reasons for performing a cesarean:

→ *An absolute indication* means there is no question or doubt about whether a C-section is required. It is definite.
→ *A relative indication* means you *may* need to have a cesarean delivery.
  - There are reasons you'll know about before labor begins that may lead to an eventual cesarean.
  - Occasionally, possible reasons for a C-section are discovered only once labor begins.

REASONS FOR A CESAREAN

The following chart explains the categories of cesarean sections: why you might need one, or whether it will absolutely be scheduled.

Definitely a Cesarean

Placenta previa
- ✤ The placenta is situated between the baby and your cervix.
- ✤ A "total placenta previa" means the placenta is completely blocking the baby's exit from the womb.
- ✤ A C-section is necessary.
- ✤ A "partial placenta previa" may not be an absolute indication. It depends how much of the placenta is blocking the baby.

Placenta abruptio
- ✤ Partial or complete detachment of the placenta from the uterine wall before the baby is born.
- ✤ Risk to the mother: hemorrhaging.
- ✤ Risk to the baby: interruption of his oxygen supply.

Prolapsed cord
- ✤ The umbilical cord slips down in front of the baby's presenting part.
- ✤ Vaginal delivery would compress the cord, cutting off the baby's oxygen supply.

Maybe a Cesarean

INDICATIONS *BEFORE* LABOR

Rh incompatibility	✤ When a woman with Rh negative blood is pregnant with an Rh positive baby.
	✤ Vaginal delivery increases the chance that your blood will mix with the baby's.
	✤ This would build up antibodies in your blood that are deadly to your next baby.
Breech birth	✤ If the baby is in a breech (buttocks-first) position or transverse lie (sideways position).
	✤ Vaginal delivery could be hazardous to the baby, who might get stuck halfway out.
Previous cesarean	✤ Depends on the reason for the previous C-section.
	✤ Depends what kind of incision was made before.
Postmaturity	✤ Tests indicate the baby is at least two weeks past the due date.
	✤ Test show the placenta is no longer providing sufficient support for the baby.
Maternal disease	✤ In some cases of diabetes, kidney disease, and toxemia the mother's health may be endangered by the stress of labor.
	✤ Mothers with herpes simplex virus II who have active vaginal sores at the time of delivery can infect their baby in the birth canal.

Maybe a Cesarean

Cephalopelvic disproportion	✦ The baby's head is too large to fit through the mother's pelvis.
Mother over 40	✦ A woman having her first baby past the age of forty may lack the elasticity in her pelvis to give birth vaginally.
Fetal distress	✦ This refers to distress that continues after changes in position and other corrective measures designed to improve oxygen supply to the fetus.
Ruptured membranes	✦ Labor does not start (or is prolonged) after membranes break.
	✦ The infection rate rises if a woman has not given birth within twenty-four hours after her membranes rupture.

THE OPERATION

Preparation

→ You will check into the hospital two hours prior to the operation or the night before.

→ Samples of your blood and urine will be taken.

→ You will be shaved from your belly button down through the upper portion of your pubic hair.

→ If you check in at night you may be given a sleeping pill to calm you and help you get a good night's sleep.

→ A sedative before the operation may be given by injection.

    • Discuss possible medications with the anesthesiologist beforehand.

    • Drugs reach the baby and make him groggy on delivery, which can delay sucking and bonding.

    • You can refuse this medication.

→ A catheter will be inserted into your bladder. This plastic tube that drains your bladder during the operation is painlessly inserted.

How the operation is performed
→ There are two kinds of cesareans.
→ A *classical* incision is vertical, with a longitudinal cut made on top of the uterus.
 - It is the quickest way to cut a cesarean and may be done if speed is essential in an emergency.
 - A classical incision is more difficult to repair. It has a 2 percent chance of rupture in future pregnancies.
→ A *transverse* incision (also called a "bikini cut") is a horizontal incision made below your pubic hairline.
 - It is made at the bottom of the uterus.
 - It's easy to repair and unlikely to rupture in the future.
→ A cesarean takes forty-five minutes to one hour.
→ From the beginning of the skin incision to delivery is the shortest part of the operation: five to six minutes.
→ The repair of the uterine and abdominal walls takes the most time.
→ After the baby is delivered the placenta is removed.
→ An oxytocic drug is given to encourage your uterus to contract.
 - These contractions can be painful; you may need to use your breathing techniques.
→ If stitches are used they will need to be removed between five and seven days after surgery.
→ Some doctors close the skin with metal clips that can be removed in a week or less.

Medication during surgery
→ An epidural is the anesthesia most often used (see page 215 for information on medications during labor).
→ After delivery the mother is often given a drug called Duramorf, a morphine drug that stays in a woman's body about twenty-four hours, reducing postoperative pain.
→ A woman has to be watched carefully for a twenty-four-hour period after the drug is administered.
→ When the anesthetic begins wearing off in the recovery room you will become aware of the pain from the incision.
→ If you are given pain medication you may become nauseated.
 - Throwing up is painful after abdominal surgery.
 - If you are prone to nausea ask your doctor before surgery about receiving an antiemetic drug with pain medication to prevent nausea.

Emotional aspects of a cesarean

→ Some women have negative feelings about a cesarean.

→ It is important to keep your perspective. The most important thing is that a healthy baby is being born.

→ If your doctor tells you it's necessary ahead of time:
- Get a second opinion about whether you need a cesarean.
- This eliminates possible doubts later that the cesarean could have been avoided.

→ Ask about hospital policies for allowing the father into the operating room.
- You may feel lonely and scared and in need of your partner's support.
- Having him there may reduce his feelings of inadequacy from being excluded from the birth process.

→ Lowering the screen to let you see the baby being born will help you connect to the baby you've been carrying inside.

→ Unless the baby needs immediate medical attention ask if you can hold her for a little while after birth.

→ Breast-feeding on the delivery table or in the recovery room is possible if the baby is fine. Discuss it with your doctor beforehand.

→ Bonding immediately at birth is particularly crucial for cesarean mothers and babies because the natural birth process has been interrupted.

→ It is routine for many hospitals to place a cesarean baby in the intensive-care nursery or central nursery after birth.
- If it isn't possible to keep a healthy baby with you, make every effort to have the baby released to your room as soon as possible.
- Unless there are medical problems, there is no reason why you should be separated from your baby.

WHAT TO EXPECT IN THE
FIRST DAYS AFTER CESAREAN

The IV
- The IV is kept in for twenty-four to forty-eight hours after surgery, depending on your condition.

The catheter
- The catheter that emptied your bladder during surgery will be removed within twenty-four hours.

Bowel movements
- Bowel movements may be difficult after surgery.
- Straining is uncomfortable after an abdominal incision: it's important to keep your stool soft.
- Ask your doctor about taking a stool softener (often prescribed routinely).

Abdominal pain
- This pain will lessen within seven to ten days.
- Involuntary movements of your stomach muscles may hurt.
- Hold your hands or a pillow pressed against the incision when you laugh or cough.

The scar
- The scar can be itchy.
- It's also common for it to ooze a little.
- If the stitches are nonabsorbable they will be removed about a week after surgery.

Nursing
- Nursing may be uncomfortable at first.
- Try putting a pillow over your stomach.

Avoid stair-climbing
- For the first week or two, avoid stairs if it is possible.
- Climbing stairs puts a strain on your stomach muscles and can increase incision pain.

Avoid lifting
- Lifting *anything* forces you to use the abdominal muscles, which have been cut.
- The less you strain that area, the faster it can recover.
- Wait to lift things until fifteen days after surgery, when the incision heals and becomes stronger.

VAGINAL BIRTH AFTER CESAREAN (VBAC)

* It was once believed: "Once a C-section, always a C-section."
* The American College of Obstetricians and Gynecologists (ACOG) has declared a VBAC perfectly safe for mother and baby, even if the mother has had two or three cesareans.
* A VBAC is encouraged unless there is a current medical indication for a repeat cesarean.

The new ACOG guidelines for VBAC

→ There should be only one baby with an estimated weight of less than eight pounds eight ounces.
→ The previous cesarean should have been transverse: VBAC is not safe with a previous classical (vertical) incision.
→ There should be continuous electronic monitoring of fetal heart rate and uterine activity throughout labor.
→ When you arrive for delivery your blood should be typed and screened for irregular antibodies.

CONDITIONS FOR A VBAC

✤ Previous low transverse incision (bikini cut)
✤ Normal pregnancy
✤ Delivery within twelve to twenty-four hours after rupture of membranes
✤ Willing to avoid pain medications (or use minimal amounts) to have full feeling in case of pain due to rupture
✤ Avoidance of pitocin to induce labor; pitocin (or other forms of oxytocin) to be used only with an internal fetal monitor
✤ Understanding that general anesthetic may be used if a serious problem develops requiring an immediate cesarean

Making the decision to have a VBAC

→ Finding a supportive doctor is very important. Word of mouth is one of the best ways: ask friends and childbirth educators, or contact local childbirth organizations.

→ Accept the reality that no matter what you decide, there is always a chance that another cesarean may become necessary.

→ Be aware of the benefits of a VBAC:

   ❧ Eliminating operative and postoperative complications, reducing your hospital stay.

   ❧ Infection rates for mothers after vaginal delivery are much lower than those after cesarean births.

   ❧ Labor can be beneficial to the baby, readying her lungs for life outside the womb.

→ Discuss VBAC with your partner and your doctor.

→ Respect your own feelings about what is best for you and your baby; don't let yourself be pressured one way or the other.

12.
Special Needs and Complications

As we all know, nature is not perfect and not all pregnancies are flawless. Fortunately, there is only a small percentage of pregnancies or births in which things do go wrong. However, there is no need to read this section and perhaps alarm yourself unnecessarily. What follows is designed for those couples who have been identified as having particular risks or problems, to give them information and support.

EMERGENCY CHILDBIRTH

* This is not intended as a do-it-yourself birth guide.
* This is an outline of what to do if the baby wants to be born before you reach the hospital or the doctor or midwife reaches you.

If the urge to push comes
→ Try to avoid pushing.
→ Remain calm and assess the situation.
→ If you are home call the paramedics.
→ If you are driving to the hospital and the urge to push is too strong, stop the car.
  - If possible, cover the backseat and car floor with a layer of newspapers.
  - Lie across the backseat and deliver the baby into your husband's hands.

If you see a piece of gray-blue shiny cord
→ Call the paramedics immediately—*before anything else.*
→ Get into the knee-chest position.
  - Get on your knees with your head down and your buttocks in the air.
  - This reduces pressure on the cord.
→ If the cord is still protruding in a knee-chest position:
  - Cover it with a *very* clean towel.
  - But *do not put pressure* on the cord.
→ This is a *prolapsed cord,* which comes out of the vagina before anything else.
→ This cuts off the baby's oxygen supply and can be *fatal.*
→ A prolapsed cord means you *must* have a cesarean delivery.
→ Stay in the knee-chest position until the paramedics arrive.
→ Remain in this position even on the way to the hospital.

Never hold your legs together.
→ Do not let anyone else hold your legs together to delay the birth.
→ This can cause *brain damage* to your baby.

Put clean towels or newspapers under you.
→ If there's time.

Ease the baby out with contractions.
→ A baby coming out this fast will not require much pushing.
→ There is more chance that your vagina will tear if you push along with the force of the uterus.
→ Pant lightly with each contraction.

Deliver the head slowly.
→ It is best to push it out *between* contractions.
→ Your mate should support the perineum (the area between your vagina and anus) with a very clean towel.
→ Putting the heel of his hand over the area avoids tearing the perineum.
→ Support the baby's head as she is born.

Never pull on the baby's head to get it out.
→ Pulling can cause permanent injuries.
→ If the head is still covered by membranes:
   ᴥ Remove the membranes using fingernails, a pin, or any sharp instrument.
   ᴥ Be very careful not to scratch the baby's head.
   ᴥ Dip the tool in alcohol before using it, if there is time.
→ The membranes have to be removed in order for the baby to breathe.

Once the head is out
→ Check with fingers to feel if the cord is wrapped around the baby's neck.
→ Loosen the cord gently. Pull it over the baby's head or loosen it enough for the body to deliver through the loop.
→ The head will naturally turn to one side to allow the shoulders to rotate.
→ At this point you should push with the next contraction to deliver the shoulders.

Do not pull on the baby.
→ Support her whole body as she is born.
→ Do not do anything with the umbilical cord.

After the baby is born

→ Wrap him in a clean blanket.

→ Keep the head covered to prevent heat loss.

→ Wrap him with the uncut umbilical cord (and the placenta, when it delivers).

→ Hold the baby with his head lower than his body.

    ➴ His face should be down or to the side to allow mucus in his nose and lungs to drain.

    ➴ Do *not* wipe out the inside of his mouth.

→ The normal color of the baby at birth is blue. He "pinks up" in the first minute as oxygen enters his body. The hands and feet take longer.

→ Get the baby to the hospital for examination immediately.

Put the baby to your breast.

→ Do this only if the umbilical cord is long enough to reach without pulling on the baby's navel.

→ Even if the baby does not want to suck, being at your breast will comfort him.

→ Sucking will contract your uterus and help expel the placenta.

After the placenta is born

→ Wrap the placenta with the baby until you reach the hospital.

→ Massage your uterus *firmly* with deep circular motions within the limits of comfort.

    ➴ Push down two or three inches below your navel and rub.

    ➴ This helps the uterus contract and prevents bleeding.

→ It is normal for about two cups of blood to come out when the placenta delivers and for a few minutes afterward.

TESTS FOR COMPLICATIONS

Ultrasound
- Produces a picture of the baby in the uterus without the hazards of X-rays.
- Is used before amniocentesis to pinpoint the location of the baby and the placenta.
- Identifies disorders such as:
  - hydrocephalus (fluid on the brain)
  - ectopic pregnancy (pregnancy in the fallopian tube rather than the uterus)
- There is minimal risk to the mother or baby.

Amniocentesis
- A painless needle is inserted in your abdomen.
- Some amniotic fluid is extracted for examination.
- This is the most reliable test for determining the exact age of the baby.
- Also used to see whether a baby is past due and should be delivered.
- This test is not risk-free; there is a small chance of infection or premature labor (i.e., miscarriage).

FETAL MONITOR TESTING

The fetal heart monitor (FHM) consists of two belts put around your belly that measure the fetal heart rate (FHR) as well as the contractions of your uterus. The results are printed out on a video screen and simultaneously on paper.

Oxytocin challenge test
- An OCT is done at thirty-one to forty-four weeks (before labor begins naturally).
- A weak oxytocin (usually pitocin) is used to start contractions.
- Uterine contractions are induced to measure how the baby's heart can handle the stress of labor.
- A "positive OCT" (the baby's heart is stressed by contractions) indicates immediate delivery, usually by cesarean.
- A "negative OCT" shows no abnormal fetal heart rate changes in response to contractions.

MISCARRIAGE

What causes a pregnancy to fail?

- A miscarriage early in the pregnancy occurs as often as one in ten pregnancies.
- Miscarriage happens most often in first pregnancies.
- This is nature's way of discarding a defective embryo; it often occurs without the woman's even knowing she was pregnant.
- Within the first twenty-eight days a miscarriage appears just like a heavy menstrual period.

REASONS FOR MISCARRIAGE

- ❖ A defective sperm or egg is the most common reason.
- ❖ A hormonal problem in the mother is another cause.
- ❖ Mother and father have similar types of HLAs (human leukocyte antigens, a component of blood), which may cause a higher chance of miscarriage, usually around the twelfth week.
- ❖ Ordinary tap water may contribute to miscarriage, even if your area isn't considered polluted. (Consider using bottled, distilled water in your childbearing years.)
- ❖ Diabetes (see page 249).
- ❖ Physical problems with your uterus or cervix.
- ❖ "Recurrent miscarriage" is three or more miscarriages occurring early in pregnancy. This could be caused by: *t-mycoplasma virus* (which has no symptoms but can be treated with antibiotics), *thyroid or endocrine imbalance, poor nutrition,* or *vitamin deficiencies.*

SIGNS OF MISCARRIAGE

✤ If you're bleeding (it may not be heavy) with or without cramplike pain.

✤ Staining or bleeding with severe pain or pain that lasts more than a day.

✤ Go to bed right away and call your doctor.

✤ In some cases the pain may disappear and the pregnancy will continue.

✤ If you are miscarrying the cramps and bleeding will worsen.

✤ Don't take any alcohol or medications.

✤ Collect any signs of a miscarriage in a clean container; this may be upsetting but it can be used to determine the cause of the miscarriage.

✤ A pelvic examination will show whether you are having a miscarriage or whether the pregnancy can be saved.

✤ **WARNING:** If you are bleeding heavily enough to soak several sanitary pads in an hour or the pain is unbearable, get emergency medical attention.

WHEN CAN YOU GET PREGNANT AGAIN?

✤ Ask your doctor's advice on when it's advisable to attempt another pregnancy.

✤ If tests show you miscarried because of a defective fetus you can usually try again right after your next period.

✤ Some doctors say it's safe to have intercourse as soon as your cervix has closed: four to six weeks.

✤ Some doctors say wait three months and pay special attention to your diet and general health.

✤ If no reason is found for the miscarriage a doctor may recommend a six-month wait, hoping the unknown cause will correct itself.

✤ If the blood tests show you the miscarriage was caused by a hormonal deficiency your doctor may prescribe progesterone.

Coping with a miscarriage

→ A miscarriage can affect couples in different ways.

→ A woman's reaction can include crying, not eating, and difficulties in sleeping.

→ A man may react differently than his wife, yet a woman should not mistake her husband's lack of tears as an indication that he doesn't care.

→ Anticipate that you will feel grief.

→ Some of the normal reactions will include: loneliness, depression, guilt, anger, irritability, insomnia, and the inability to get through your normal tasks in a day.

ECTOPIC PREGNANCY

What is an ectopic pregnancy?
- Ectopic pregnancy occurs when the egg is fertilized in the fallopian tube: instead of passing into the uterus it remains and grows in the tube.
- This is dangerous if the pregnancy continues, because the tube will burst.
- A pregnancy test and physical examination can determine whether you have an ectopic pregnancy.
- Call your doctor immediately if you suspect you are pregnant and have any of the following symptoms:
  - Vaginal bleeding
  - Pain in the lower abdomen (often on one side)
  - Weakness and/or fainting
- Ectopic pregnancies are very rare.

Treatment
- Surgery must be performed to remove the fertilized egg.
- Sometimes a fallopian tube can be rebuilt; otherwise it may have to be removed.
- Removal of a fallopian tube reduces your chances of conceiving again since you're left with only one tube.
- You can have a normal pregnancy the next time, although there is a 15 percent chance of another ectopic pregnancy.

DIABETES IN PREGNANCY

Risks
- Your risk for complications increases depending on how early in your life you got diabetes and for how many years you've had the disease.
- A diabetic pregnancy can cause birth defects, usually in the first five to eight weeks, when you may not even know you're pregnant.
- Insulin-dependent diabetics have a greater risk in pregnancy.

NOTE: Women who develop diabetes *during* pregnancy *do not* have an increased risk of pregnancy complications.

Prevention

→ Good health care before pregnancy can increase the chance of a healthy baby.

→ You must eat regularly to keep your blood glucose stable.

→ A high-fiber diet may lower your need for insulin.

→ Babies of diabetics are at risk in the final weeks of pregnancy.
  - They can't go safely to term.
  - The best delivery time is usually by the thirty-sixth or thirty-seventh week.

→ Depending on what tests indicate, the baby is delivered anywhere from three to six weeks before the calculated due date, either by induced labor or cesarean.

How to handle the problem of diabetes

→ You need two doctors working together: an obstetrician who specializes in high-risk pregnancy plus an expert in diabetes.

→ Frequent trips to the doctor may be necessary since normal pregnancy hormones interfere with insulin.

→ Get in good control of your blood glucose before you get pregnant.

→ Tight control of blood sugar levels can usually be achieved with a strict diet combined with a program that teaches you to adjust your insulin dose and monitor your blood glucose level.

→ Exercise should be planned with medical supervision.

→ Moderate exercise may give you more energy and can help stabilize your blood sugar.

TOXEMIA

Why does it happen?
- The cause of this complication is not fully understood. (However, it is *not* caused by gaining too much weight, as was previously thought.)
- Poor nutrition (in particular, insufficient protein) is linked to toxemia.
- The best prevention is a well-balanced diet with foods high in protein.
- Symptoms include: rapid weight gain, severe swelling of hands and face, headaches, a rise in blood pressure, protein in the urine, and vision disturbance.

Risks
- Toxemia is uncommon. It usually happens in the last trimester.
- It is not a cause for alarm if you're getting regular medical care.
- Toxemia in the second trimester is very rare and extremely dangerous to the mother and baby.
- Toxemia can affect the baby's development because the placenta does not function as well. The results can be a small-for-date baby or fetal death.
- Labor is induced early in some cases of toxemia.

HYPERTENSION (HIGH BLOOD PRESSURE)

Risks
- If you have high blood pressure before getting pregnant you're considered high-risk.
- A low-salt diet, increased rest, and close medical observation should keep things under control.

→ If you have any of the following along with an increase of blood pressure, you have a condition called *pre-eclampsia.*
   ◆ Sudden weight gain (more than three pounds a week in the second trimester or two pounds a week in the third).
   ◆ Protein in your urine.
   ◆ Swelling from water retention in your hands, face, and ankles.
→ If pre-eclampsia isn't treated early it can progress to *eclampsia,* which is a more serious threat to mother and child.
→ Pre-eclampsia is more common in first pregnancies. It may be linked to poor nutrition.

Helpful hints
→ Temporary high blood pressure that develops during pregnancy is not considered dangerous and disappears after delivery.
→ High blood pressure in the first two trimesters will require extra medical supervision.
→ When pre-eclampsia is diagnosed the doctor may try treating you at home, although hospitalization with partial or total bed rest and medication may be required.
→ Proper medical treatment will assure your health and that of the baby.

ASTHMA

Risks
→ A severe asthmatic condition does mean a higher-risk pregnancy, but you can practically eliminate the risk with good medical supervision.
→ You have to be able to deliver oxygen regularly to the baby—an asthma attack cuts off the baby's oxygen supply.
→ Treat an asthma attack immediately with prescribed medication so you won't reduce the baby's oxygen.
→ One third of asthmatic conditions get worse (usually after the first trimester), one third are not affected, and one third actually improve.

Prevention
→ Try to avoid the factors that can trigger asthma.
→ Exercise can trigger asthma; before exerting yourself take the medications prescribed by your doctor.
→ Last-trimester breathlessness is normal for all pregnant women but can make asthma flare-ups worse.
→ A tendency to allergies and asthma is inherited; you should try to breast-feed for at least six months to delay allergic reactions in your child.

How to handle the problem
→ Find an internist and/or an allergist to work with your ob/gyn.
→ Doctors believe that asthma should be treated as aggressively during pregnancy as if you weren't pregnant; the medication poses less of a threat than an untreated asthma attack.
→ Use only drugs your doctor has prescribed for use during pregnancy and only exactly as indicated.

VAGINAL INFECTIONS

- Vaginal infections are common during pregnancy because the hormonal changes make your vagina prone to yeastlike fungi.
- If you have a vaginal discharge that is yellowish, greenish, very thick, foul-smelling, and/or you have burning, itchiness, soreness, and redness, see your doctor for treatment.
- Your doctor will do a vaginal culture to see what kind of infection you have.
- Simple yeast infections are easily treated and have no ill effect on the baby.
- If your infection is caused by the "monilia yeast," your doctor will treat it with medication so that you don't infect your baby, who would get thrush from it during birth.
- You may continue to get yeast infections during pregnancy, although the condition will stop afterward.

Helpful hints
→ Doctors usually treat vaginal infections with suppositories or creams inserted with an applicator.

→ Careful personal hygiene is important (after going to the bathroom remember to wipe toward the back, away from your vagina).

→ Taking 500 mg. of vitamin C may increase the acidity of the vagina, making it unfriendly for the growth of yeast, but check with your doctor first.

→ Boric acid baths: for every six inches of water put three tablespoons of boric acid (from a health food store or large pharmacy) in the bathtub. Soak for ten minutes.

→ Take boric acid tablets. Check with your obstetrician about whether you can take 500 mg. boric acid tablets three times a day with food.

→ Decrease sweets, especially refined sugar.

→ If the doctor says the infection can be passed on sexually, abstain from sex until both partners are free of symptoms (the man can experience irritation or burning on urination).

SEXUALLY TRANSMITTED DISEASES (STDs)

Syphilis

Risks
- ✤ Can cause miscarriage any time after the fourth month.
- ✤ Baby can be stillborn (one quarter of syphilis-infected babies) or die soon after birth (one third of babies already infected).
- ✤ Babies can have abnormalities of bones, teeth, nose, and blindness or deafness.
- ✤ Nervous system damage and delayed brain damage may occur.

Prevention
- ✤ Routine testing at the first prenatal exam.
- ✤ Early diagnosis and treatment will cure infection in the unborn baby.
- ✤ Taking antibiotics before the eighteenth week keeps the disease from crossing the placenta and infecting the baby.

Gonorrhea

Risks
- ✤ Causes eye infection in newborns that leads to blindness.
- ✤ You can have gonorrhea without suspecting it and without any symptoms.
- ✤ It often cannot be detected even by repeated tests before delivery.

Prevention
- ✤ Routine testing at the first prenatal exam.
- ✤ If the disease is discovered it can be treated immediately with antibiotics.
- ✤ All babies' eyes are medicated with antibiotic ointment at birth as a precaution.

Chlamydia

Risks
- ✤ The most common STD, so you should be tested early in pregnancy.
- ✤ Like gonorrhea, it can cause infertility when left untreated.
- ✤ The baby can get pneumonia or eye infections.

Prevention
- ✤ Prenatal antibiotic treatment can prevent infection of your baby.
- ✤ It can also be treated in the newborn if it goes undetected in the mother.

HERPES

Risks

→ Active lesions in the vagina or cervix at the time of birth will infect 50 percent of newborns during vaginal delivery.

→ Babies born with herpes will have severe nerve and/or eye damage or will die.

→ Herpes affects up to twenty million Americans and there is no cure for it yet.

→ Either the mother or her partner can transmit the disease to the baby, but it is preventable with medical supervision.

Prevention

→ Get frequent examinations from your obstetrician before you conceive or early in your pregnancy.

→ If you or your partner have an active infection, avoid sex.

→ Keep very clean, take a bath or shower daily, and always wash your hands with soap and water after using the toilet.

→ Take a shower or wash your hands after sex.

→ Wear only cotton underpants, preferably ones that are not tight.

Helpful hints

→ From about the thirty-fifth week have your obstetrician examine you weekly to make sure that herpes has not recurred in the birth canal.

→ If you do have herpes lesions at the time of delivery the baby must be delivered by cesarean before the membranes rupture (or within four hours after they do) to prevent infection.

BREECH BIRTH

* The breech position is when your baby is positioned with his buttocks leading.
* Only 3 percent of births are breach.
* In less than 1 percent of births a baby is in some other unusual position.

DIFFERENT TYPES OF
BREECH POSITIONS

Complete
❖ Baby is cross-legged in the bottom of the uterus.

Frank
❖ His legs are straight up with his feet near his face.

Footling
❖ A rare position with one or both feet coming first.

Other positions that can cause complications are:

Posterior vertex
❖ The baby faces your abdomen instead of your tailbone.

❖ If baby does not rotate before birth the doctor may rotate head with forceps.

Transverse lie
❖ The baby is lying sideways in your uterus.

❖ Unless he can be turned you will need a cesarean.

CAUSES FOR A
BREECH PRESENTATION

❖ A small or premature baby

❖ A large baby who may not have enough room to settle head-down into your pelvis

❖ Excess amniotic fluid, which allows the baby to float around instead of engaging in your pelvis

❖ Multiple pregnancy

❖ Placenta previa (placenta presenting before the baby).

❖ Uterine tumors

❖ A hydrocephalic baby with water on the brain, making the head oversize

Dangers of a breech presentation

- Because there are so many risks in a breech presentation the common practice is to deliver all breeches by cesarean section.
- Labor can be longer or simply not progress because the buttocks are not as effective as the head in opening the birth canal.
- Prolapsed cord occurs ten times as often in breech births.
- The cord can be compressed in its passage through the pelvis, cutting off the baby's oxygen supply.
- Fractures, dislocations, and nerve damage are more common in vaginal breech deliveries because of the complications in getting the baby out.

Vaginal delivery with a breech presentation

→ The National Institutes of Health (NIH) has found that there are conditions when a vaginal delivery should be considered an acceptable obstetrical choice for a breech birth.
- Anticipated weight of baby is less than eight pounds.
- Normal pelvic shape and size.
- Frank breech presentation without a hyperextended head.

→ If you wish to attempt a vaginal delivery it is important to find a doctor who is experienced in vaginal breech presentation delivery.

→ You will be considered a high-risk pregnancy: some hospitals will have an anesthesiologist in attendance so that a cesarean can be done immediately if it becomes necessary.

→ Once you are in labor if there is any fetal distress, or labor does not progress, the doctor will perform a cesarean.

→ Gravity is the greatest help during labor in breech and posterior presentations, so you should sit as upright as possible.

→ "Piper forceps" are a special kind of gentle forceps used for delivering breech babies. They are not used to pull the baby out but only to keep his head flexed down.

→ The doctor may try to rotate the baby from outside before labor begins, although many babies return to the breech position.

→ If you know you are having a breech birth you can try the following exercise around the thirtieth week of pregnancy and continue for at least four to six weeks:
- Lie with your back on the floor and your pelvis raised nine to twelve inches off the floor, resting on three large pillows.
- Your knees should be bent and your feet flat on the floor.
- If it's not very comfortable, you are doing it right.
- Do this twice a day on an empty stomach and stay in position for ten minutes each time.
- Some babies have been encouraged to shift to a head-first presentation by this method.

TWINS

Risks
- There is a greater chance of premature labor and premature babies have a greater risk of complications.
- There is increased risk of toxemia: you should eat a lot of high-quality protein and get plenty of rest.
- A greater proportion of sluggish labor occurs with twins because the uterus has been overdistended during pregnancy and contractions are weaker.
- Unusual presentation of the babies is common, with one baby head-first and the second breech.
- The twins take up more room and demand more from your circulatory system, which can increase minor discomforts.
- The likelihood of producing twins is a hereditary tendency.
- Women aged thirty-five to forty years old are three times more likely to have twins than a woman under twenty.
- Women who become pregnant soon after going off birth control pills also have a higher chance of bearing twins.
- Because half of all twins arrive prematurely, they have a greater risk of underdeveloped lungs.
- Risks to mothers include increased incidence of anemia, high blood pressure, and hemorrhage after delivery.
- Because the birth is more complicated, about half of all twins are delivered by cesarean section.

Identical twins
- Identical twins are the result of one egg fertilized by one sperm.
- Once the egg is fertilized it splits into two, resulting in two babies of the same sex and exactly alike in skin, hair, and eye color.
- Identical twins are much less common.

Fraternal twins
- Fraternal twins are the result of two different eggs fertilized by two different spermatozoa.
- Fraternal twins can be of different sexes and blood groups and are nonidentical.
- Nonidentical twins are the most common.

POLYHYDRAMNIOS
(EXCESS AMNIOTIC FLUID)

What it means and how it affects your baby

- The normal amount of amniotic fluid is one liter (slightly over one quart).
- More than about two quarts of fluid is considered polyhydramnios.
- The condition is often associated with diabetes, toxemia, or multiple births, but the cause is not known.
- Polyhydramnios can cause greater than normal edema (swelling) of the legs and vulva, difficulty breathing and sleeping, indigestion, heartburn, and constipation.
- The condition can cause premature labor because your uterus is overstretched.
- Unusual position of the baby is common because she can float around more.
- There is a relatively high prenatal mortality rate associated with this condition; the rate increases as the amount of fluid increases.
- If you have a severe form of this condition you should see an obstetrician who specializes in high-risk pregnancies.

PROBLEMS WITH THE PLACENTA

Placenta previa
- The placenta is situated low down in the uterus instead of at the top and blocks the cervix so the baby cannot exit.
- The symptom is vaginal bleeding during the last trimester.
- If the doctor feels the placenta blocking the cervix he will perform a cesarean.
- If he cannot feel any placenta or only a sliver of it, then he will rupture the membranes and induce labor.
- About 60 percent of women with placenta previa have cesareans.

Placenta abruptio
- The premature separation of part or all of the placenta from the uterine wall.
- This normally occurs after the birth of the baby.
- This condition is more common in women who have had five or six babies.
- Symptoms include vaginal bleeding accompanied by abdominal pain in the last weeks of pregnancy.
- A cesarean birth may be necessary.

FORCEPS DELIVERY

* Forceps are large curved tongs that are slipped inside your vagina on either side of the baby's head so the doctor can pull the baby out by her head.
* Forceps can save a baby's life in a complicated delivery but no other country uses them for as many normal births as does the United States.

THE THREE KINDS OF FORCEPS DELIVERY

High forceps	✤ Performed very rarely.
	✤ The cesarean section has replaced high forceps as a way to deliver a baby that will not descend.
Mid or low forceps	✤ Used only when absolutely necessary because it involves inserting the forceps quite high and exerting a lot of pull on the baby.
	✤ May be necessary if anesthesia has made it impossible for you to push the baby out.
Outlet or perineal forceps	✤ Is commonly used when the baby's head is visible at the perineum, or his scalp can be clearly seen if the lips of your vagina are spread open.
	✤ The forceps are used to lift the baby out of the vagina.

The usual reasons for a forceps delivery

* To speed up second-stage labor if there is severe fetal distress.
* If the cord is wrapped tightly around the baby's neck or the cord prolapses.
* In case of unusual presentations.
* To shorten a very long second stage of labor.
* If regional anesthesia doesn't allow you to push the baby out.

Risks

* Complications of forceps delivery are rare.
* The most common problem is that the forceps can bruise the baby's head, but it clears up in a few days.
* On rare occasions the pressure of the forceps can cause intracranial bleeding and damage to the infant's facial nerves.

PREMATURE LABOR

What is considered "premature" and how is it a problem?
- Premature labor is calculated on the baby's birth weight instead of the length of pregnancy.
- When a newborn weighs less than five and a half pounds it is considered a premature infant.
- Ordinarily a five-and-a-half-pound baby is four weeks before its due date. At that weight it has more complications, particularly with underdeveloped lungs.

How to stop premature labor
- → Doctors can use medication to attempt to halt labor once it has started.
- → There are side effects to these drugs: hypotension, dizziness, and nausea.
- → An intravenous alcohol solution given over several hours is also thought to stop labor.
- → If the membranes rupture prematurely but contractions do not begin a woman may be placed flat in bed in the hospital to halt the onset of labor until she's closer to her due date.

What to expect if your baby is premature
- A premie's first hours are crucial. If they're born in a hospital with a neonatal intensive care unit they generally do better.
- Underdeveloped lungs are the main problem with premies; many are placed in a ventilator, a device that mechanically expands and contracts the newborn's tiny lungs until they develop sufficiently.
- Premies have a greater chance of becoming jaundiced because their underdeveloped livers are not functioning properly.

Feelings about having a premie
- → Anxiety is the primary emotion you will feel.
- → Most premature babies do survive, but hearing pessimistic remarks in the first hours of her life can cause you anxiety.
- → Insure that the baby's father is included in all discussions about the baby's condition.
- → You need to have your partner with you as much as possible.

→ A premie bears little resemblance to a full-term newborn: you may feel frightened at the sight of your baby, who will most likely be scrawny and naked with tubes coming out of her nose.

→ The sight of the equipment might increase your anxiety so ask the nurse assigned to your baby to explain all the contraptions.

→ Get confidence and lessons from the nurses in holding, feeding, and diapering your baby.

→ Try to minimize your separation from the baby to whatever extent you can.

→ Make an effort to establish eye-to-eye contact with the baby—this gives you reinforcing feedback and is important to maternal-infant bonding.

→ Breast-feeding is excellent because it gives you a sense of accomplishment.

→ If the baby is not yet strong enough to suck, you can express breast milk and feed the baby through a nose tube.

→ Bonding with your baby is very important; stay involved in your child's progress and emphasize plenty of close contact and touching.

PART IV

YOU AND YOUR NEW BABY

Simply Wonderful

13.

The New Baby

What's Normal,
What's Not

Many new parents in America have never been
around little babies until they have their own.
This chapter lets you know which "strange"
things about a newborn are actually normal!
This chapter also helps you to make many of the
important early decisions that can be confusing.

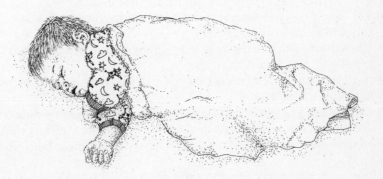

YOUR NEWBORN'S APPEARANCE

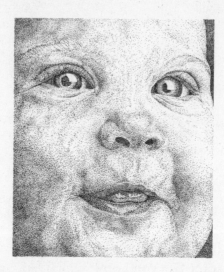

Don't expect your newborn to look like a Gerber baby. They rarely do! Here's what's normal for many babies to look like and act like in the early weeks.

Skin

- Can be blotchy, pink, red, pale, or dry and scaly.
- White bumps on nose, cheeks, or forehead are plugged oil glands. These will come and go in the first months.
- The skin may peel for a few days after birth. (Don't pick at it, the skin comes off naturally.)
- "Newborn rash" comes from skin's supersensitivity. This rash may be in one area or all over.
- Birthmarks are common on any part of the body. They usually fade in the first year.
- Mongolian spots are irregular gray-blue or purple pigmentation in the lower back or buttocks area. They occur in African-American, Mediterranean, or Oriental infants. They will disappear by school age.
- Lanugo is a soft hair covering the baby's skin at birth. It falls out in the first weeks of life.

Head

- May be oval or odd-shaped, depending on how much pressure there was during birth.
- Soft spots of the head allow for brain growth. These close by the age of twelve to eighteen months.
- Most babies develop an "average" head of hair by the time they're eighteen months old.
- The tops of the ears may be curled down at birth. They will uncurl soon.
- The head is wobbly; it's large and the neck muscles aren't developed yet. The head always needs support in the early months.

Eyes

- Usually gray or slate-blue at birth.
- Permanent eye color comes in between six to twelve months.
- The eyes may be puffy, red, or have drainage in the first days. This is usually caused by the ointment placed in the baby's eyes at birth to prevent infection.
- A newborn's eyes are crossed because the muscles that keep both eyes pointing in the same direction aren't working yet.
- There may be a red spot or two in the baby's eye after birth. This is caused by a blood vessel that broke during delivery and will clear by itself.
- A baby can see, but can focus only up to nine inches away from his eyes.

Umbilical cord

- The cord stump should be kept dry, although you can cleanse it with alcohol.
- Keep the cord stump above the diaper and protected from rubbing.
- The cord will dry to a black hard stump and fall off in about a week. There may be some bloody drainage when this happens.
- NOTIFY THE DOCTOR OF SIGNS OF INFECTION: bleeding, redness, or odor.

External genitals

- Boys' and girls' genitals are both often swollen at birth.
- A baby girl can have discharge from the vagina that is white and mucuslike or reddish. This is a normal reaction to the hormones that were in her mother's system.

- Milk in the baby's breasts is fairly common for both boys and girls. They are influenced by the same hormones that prepare the mother's breasts to give milk. This passes in a few days.

Bowel movements

- The first bowel movement is a greenish black tarlike substance that is in the baby's intestines at birth.
- The stools change in the first days until they become yellow and pasty.
- There is no "normal" number of bowel movements for a newborn. It can be one or many and occur daily or on alternate days.
- Every baby strains, turns red in the face, and draws up his legs during the first bowel movement(s).

Circulation and temperature

- Hands and feet may look darker in color because the baby's circulation is immature and hasn't developed enough to carry warm blood to the ends of these limbs.
- A newborn's heating system is inefficient. Be aware of the baby's temperature.
- Cool hands and feet and a warm belly means he's at a good temperature.

Newborn reflexes

- A newborn tends to jump at noises and may tremble. This is just a sign that the baby's reflex system is adjusting.
- The "rooting reflex" causes the baby to turn his head toward anything that touches his cheek. This helps a baby find food by rooting around for the mother's nipple.
- The baby's hearing is impaired during the first few days because the middle part of the eardrum is full of amniotic fluid.

CRYING

* Crying is a baby's way of expressing discomfort or hunger. It may also be a way of "letting off steam."
* If you check his diaper and feed him and burp him and he still cries when you put him back down, you have to make some decisions.

TIPS ABOUT CRYING

+ Some people set a fifteen-minute limit: they let the baby cry that long before picking her up.
+ The baby may need to cry as a way of releasing tension.
+ A baby does *not* cry as a manipulative way of getting attention.
+ You can be as responsive and indulgent as you want.
+ Responding to his crying gives the baby a sense of security.
+ Overhandling of a baby can tire him and cause crying and fussiness.
+ If your baby gets fussy from too much handling you can swaddle him, which is calming.

CIRCUMCISION

Professional opinion changes constantly about the benefits or harms of circumcising newborn boys. Talk to your pediatrician and look at the reasons for and against circumcision before making a decision.

REASONS FOR CIRCUMCISION	REASONS AGAINST CIRCUMCISION
■ May reduce chances of urinary tract infection. ■ May reduce the risk of contracting and passing on sexually transmitted diseases later in life. ■ Reduces the chance of penile cancer. ■ A circumcised penis is easier to keep clean.	■ It causes the baby pain and perhaps trauma. ■ Circumcision is the most commonly performed surgery on males in the United States, yet only 1 percent of the males in all of Europe are circumcised.

Suggestions when circumcising

→ You should wait at least twelve to twenty-four hours after birth before circumcising your baby. This allows him to have a gentle beginning in life.

→ The baby's weight should be considered. If he weighs less than six pounds you may want to delay the operation until he is larger.

→ A mother or father may want to hold the baby for the procedure. This might lessen the trauma for the infant.

JAUNDICE

Jaundice has three forms: normal, abnormal, and breast-milk jaundice (which is *very* rare).

Normal (or physiologic) jaundice

- Occurs around three to four days after birth and before the second week.
- The baby has a slight yellowing of the skin—a tinge of yellow almost like a tan.
- In this type there are no complicating factors.

Abnormal jaundice

- The baby's color is obviously jaundiced: the yellow is medium to deep.
- The jaundice occurs in conjunction with a fever or cold.
- There was oxygen deprivation in labor or the mother is diabetic.
- The way to be sure is a visit to the pediatrician, who'll decide if a blood test is needed.
- Most doctors suggest hospitalization for abnormal jaundice. You'll be separated, and that limits breast-feeding.
- Discuss reservations you have about hospitalizing your newborn. Your pediatrician may suggest alternative treatments.

Breast-milk jaundice

- Usually occurs at the beginning of the second week.
- It's probably caused by a hormone related to progesterone that's secreted in the milk.
- You may have to discontinue nursing temporarily.
- Breast-milk jaundice does not cause harm to the baby.

FACTORS THAT MAY CONTRIBUTE TO JAUNDICE

- ✤ If the baby is dehydrated.
- ✤ If the baby is too cool.
- ✤ The baby experienced a lot of bruising during birth.
- ✤ While pregnant you took aspirin, caffeine, or Valium.
- ✤ The baby is premature, which means the liver is usually immature.

THINGS YOU'LL NEED
FOR THE BABY

Baby's room

→ The baby's room should be painted with nontoxic paint. Remove old paint first. Do not repaint over old paint, because a child can get lead poisoning from flakes of old paint.

→ A cradle is cute but the baby grows out of it quickly. Don't bother buying one.

REQUIREMENTS FOR A CRIB

✤ Bars no farther apart than 2 3/8 inches (otherwise the baby's head could get stuck).

✤ A railing 26 inches higher than the lowest level of the mattress support (so the baby can't climb out).

✤ A mattress that fits snugly (to avoid baby's head's getting stuck between the mattress and crib).

✤ Smooth surfaces.

✤ Safe and sturdy hardware and a secure teething rail all the way around.

✤ A crib with one side-drop is more stable and less expensive than one in which both side rails can lower.

✤ Crib guards make it safer and softer for the baby.

✤ *Never use pillows as crib guards:* they can smother the baby and are bad for posture.

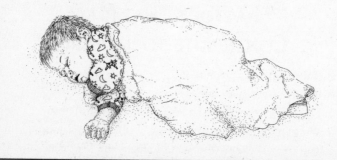

WARNING: Mesh-side cribs and playpens can be dangerous if sides are left down. Children have suffocated when they rolled into the space between the mattress and the loose mesh siding. There are now warning labels on most of these products. When buying, look for a product with no gap at all between the mattress and sides. *Never* leave a child in one of these cribs with the side down.

Basic bedding needs

- A waterproof mattress
- Two or three waterproof mattress pads
- Two quilted crib pads
- Four to six crib sheets
- Crib bumpers
- Two crib blankets or bag-type sleepers

Basic supplies

- A rectal thermometer
- Blunt baby nail scissors
- Premoistened wipe cloths
- Rubbing alcohol (to dab on the umbilical cord until it falls off)
- Baby soap and mild "no tears" shampoo
- Diaper rash ointment
- *A strap on the changing table is essential*—even if you're going to use a bureau top for changing. (Babies can fall off in the time it takes you to turn around.)
- Two pacifiers (useful when the baby won't quiet down)
- *Do not use cotton swabs* in either ears or nose (can be damaging).
- *Do not use mineral oil* on the baby (it absorbs oil-soluble vitamins through the skin).

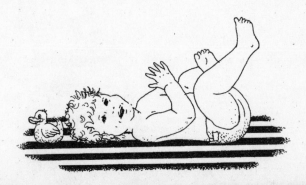

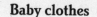

Baby clothes

- Get the six-month size in clothes for any newborn except premie.
- You will need:
  - ❧ Six to ten T-shirts
  - ❧ Four to six stretch coveralls ("onesies")
- If the baby develops a rash it may be from clothes washed in detergent containing phosphate or from fabric softener. Change to a mild infant soap like Ivory or Dreft.
- Be careful about sleepwear. The fire-retardant chemical Tris has been banned from use in sleepwear. It can cause cancer through the baby's skin.

Exercise equipment for baby

- These devices should not be used very often. They may impair development of reflexes when your child learns to fall naturally.
- Jumpers are not recommended by some doctors who say they force physical development ahead of natural timing.
- Bouncers and walkers can be dangerous if the X part of the supporting frame does not have a plastic cover to prevent babies' fingers from getting caught.
- Walkers should not tip if the child bumps into another object.

Strollers

- Should not tip if the child reaches out.
- They should have no sharp edges or scissor-type action parts that can harm fingers.

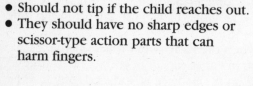

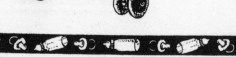

INFANT CAR SEATS

For the latest information on car seat safety call the National Child Passenger Safety Association Hotline at 1-800-424-9393.

CAR SEAT SAFETY

❖ Fasten harness or anchor straps *tightly.*	Allows child to sustain severe jolts during a collision.
❖ Always place infant facing backwards.	Child should not face forward until he or she weighs seventeen to twenty pounds and sits up well.
❖ Always secure seat with the *lap* seat belt.	If the lap belt does not fit try another seating position or get a seat belt extender.
❖ Always use the harness.	Without the harness the child can be thrown out of the car seat.
❖ Do not bundle the baby in blankets.	Bundling prevents correct position of the shoulder harness. In cold weather cut holes in one blanket and pull straps through holes.
❖ The baby's position in the seat	Flat back (no slouch) against the back of the seat. Support a small infant's head with thin blankets placed in the small of the back and on either side of the body.
❖ Always fasten the top anchor strap.	The seat can turn forward in a head-on collision if not anchored.
❖ Never ever let the child ride unsecured.	Never make any exceptions about using a car seat.

FEEDING BABY

GENERAL POINTERS ABOUT FEEDING

Begin feeding in a calm, relaxed atmosphere.

If the baby is very hungry and crying, try to calm him down before attempting feeding. If the baby is tense his stomach will be tight, his breathing will be out of rhythm, and he won't nurse or digest as well.

When you nurse, hold the baby firmly so he feels secure.

Hold his foot or bottom with a firm touch and keep his back fairly straight—he can't digest well if he's hunched over.

Feeding the baby at night

Change his diaper before you feed him so he will be clean and dry and will wake up, which allows him to nurse well.

Burping

You can burp the baby over your shoulder or with his face downward on your lap. Another position is with the baby sitting up: you support his back and head with one hand, gently moving him back and forward.

Choking

If the baby spits up, chokes, and gags, *sit him up immediately.*

If you are bottle-feeding

It is important to offer the bottle on both sides. If you always hold the baby on the same side her eye coordination can suffer.

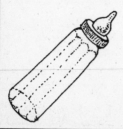

BREAST-FEEDING

Advantages to baby
→ Breast-fed babies are healthier.
      ᴥ Some studies show a greater incidence of illness in bottle-fed infants.
→ Human milk is more digestible.
→ Breast-fed babies are rarely constipated.
→ The nutrients in breast milk are more easily absorbed.
→ There is less likelihood of overfeeding when you breast-feed because the baby feeds only until he is satisfied.
→ Breast-feeding is a wonderful way to bond with your baby.

Advantages to you
→ Breast-feeding immediately after birth promotes uterine contractions. This reduces the risk of hemorrhage and returns the uterus to its pre-pregnancy size.
→ Breast-feeding is less expensive than formulas.
→ Breast-feeding is more convenient without the hassle of bottles.
→ Some experts indicate a decreased incidence of breast cancer in women who breast-fed.

Preparation for breast-feeding
→ Rub your nipples gently with a towel. This accustoms your nipples to the stimulation they'll get from the baby.
→ Pull out your nipples firmly, using oil or cream as lubricant.
→ You'll need a minimum of three nursing bras that support your breasts and protect your clothes from leaking.
→ Smaller-breasted women find that stretch bras give enough support and they can just lift the entire bra up over their breast while they're nursing.
→ Disposable nursing pads absorb any leakage. They also protect your breast from detergent residues that can irritate it.
→ Breast shields can be used to catch leaking milk.

Nutrition
→ When nursing you need an extra 500 calories and an extra 20 grams of protein a day. (This does *not* mean brownies!)
→ Continue taking a 30 to 60 mg. iron supplement during breast-feeding.

→ No oral contraceptives during breast-feeding.
→ Drink plenty of fluids in order to produce milk. You need two to three quarts of liquid a day.

Lactation consultants

→ This is a new kind of health-care provider who helps with breast-feeding difficulties.
→ A consultation lasts about an hour and a half. The consultant will check your breasts, evaluate your milk supply, and examine the baby's position and ways of sucking.
→ She can suggest techniques to correct or reduce any problems you have.

General information about breast-feeding

→ *Colostrum* is a watery or creamy yellow liquid. It comes before your milk and contains twice the protein of mature breast milk.
→ Your milk will come in within five to seven days. The colostrum provides enough nourishment until then.
→ Colostrum and breast milk provide antibodies that protect against various bacteria and viruses. This is one reason breast-fed babies are healthier.
→ You may get strong uterine contractions when you first breast-feed. Suckling releases the hormone oxytocin into your system, which makes your uterus contract.
→ *Demand feeding* is the most successful. This means that the baby nurses whenever she is hungry and will eventually settle down to a schedule of her own, not one predetermined by adults.
→ Part-time breast-feeding can work if you try not to miss more than one feeding daily in the first two months; skipping the same feeding is the key to making it work.

Sore nipples

→ Be sure to let your nipples air-dry.
→ Never keep on a wet bra or pad.
→ No nursing bra should have waterproof backing, which can cause sore nipples.
→ Vitamin A and D cream can minimize discomfort. Avoid creams containing lanolin (under investigation for possible detriment to a newborn).
→ Use ointments sparingly; they keep out the light, which is important to healing.

→ Warm dry heat is the best cure for sore nipples. Leave your breasts exposed to the air as much as possible.

→ Do not avoid nursing; this just prolongs the problem.

→ Nursing frequently avoids the breast's becoming too full. Also the baby will not get so ravenous.

→ Give the least sore breast first because the baby sucks hardest when she is hungry.

Medications and breast-feeding

Any drugs that you take while nursing will be passed on to your baby. It is important to ask your doctor and/or pharmacist if medication is safe for breast-feeding. Even aspirin can cause potential problems for your newborn.

MEDICATIONS TO AVOID WHEN BREAST-FEEDING

Drug	Effect
Analgesics *Aspirin, phenacetin, and combinations* (Alka-Seltzer, Bufferin, Cope, Excedrin, Rhinex, Vanquish)	possible bleeding
Ergotamine (antimigraine) *(Cafergot, Ergomar, Gynergan, Migral)	vomiting, diarrhea, weak pulse, unstable blood pressure, shock in 90 percent of infants
Antacids (Alka-Seltzer, Gelusil, Maalox)	possible bleeding
Antibiotics *Chloromycetin	anemia, shock, death
*Erythromycin	sensitization, allergy to drug
Erythromycin estolate (Ilosone)	hepatoxic
Symmetrel	vomiting, rash
Tetracycline	bone growth retardation
Streptomycin	nephrotoxicity
*Penicillin	possible sensitization, allergy
*Antituberculosis (Isoniazid)	mental retardation

*Especially harmful.

283

DRUG	EFFECT
Anticoagulants	
*Dicumarol	blood-clotting takes longer;
*Heparin	hemorrhage in infant
Anticonvulsants	
Primidone	mother should not nurse
Mysoline	drowsiness
Dilantin	no acute side effects, occurs in only small amounts in milk
Mysoline	causes only drowsiness in baby
Antineoplastics	
MAO inhibitors (an antihypertensive drug)	nursing should stop
Antispasmodics	
Atropine combinations	diminish milk secretion;
*(Artane, Arlidin)	heart irregularities in infant
Barbiturates	
(Amytal, Luminal, Seconal, Tuinal)	may have inducing effect on baby's liver enzymes; avoid
Nembutal	may sedate baby
Hypnotics (Doriden)	drowsiness
Chloral hydrate and combinations	drowsiness
Bromides and others (Bromural, Equanil, Phenergan, Bromo-Seltzer)	drowsiness, rash
Cardiovascular preparations	
Hypotensives and combinations with diuretics	
Ismelin	hazardous to infant
*Reserpine	increased respiratory tract secretions, cyanosis, and anorexia in infant, galactorrhea in mother
Cocaine	mother should not nurse; can lead to infant death
Cough preparations	
Potassium iodide	possible thyrotropic effect in infant, skin rash

*Especially harmful.

DRUG	EFFECT

Diuretics
(Thiazides and combinations
(Diuril, Enduron)

dehydration possible; may be harmless if taken under supervision (but manufacturers say to avoid if nursing)

Hormones
*Androgen-estrogen combinations
(Deladumone, Premarin w/ Methyltestosterone)

all estrogens cause gynecomastia and lower milk production

Estrogen
(DES, TACE)

see above

Corticoids and analgesic combinations

all corticosteroids may cause poor growth and development

Glucocorticoid anti-inflammatory combinations
(Aristocort, Cetacort lotion)

poor growth in infant

Progestins
(Depo-Provera, Gynorest, Nortulate)

lower milk production

Progestins and estrogens in combination
(Demulen, Enovid, Ortho-Novum, Ovulen)

lower milk production

Parathyroid-Dihydrotachys-terol thyroid inhibitors
*(Tapazole)

osteoporosis, bone dysgenesis, reduced thyroid activity, goiter, anemia

Laxatives
Senokot
*Dorbantyl, Dorbane

loose stool
diarrhea

Marijuana

hazard to infant

Muscle relaxants
Carosoprodol

manufacturer suggests avoidance when nursing

Valium—see "Psychotropics"

*Especially harmful.

DRUG	EFFECT
Psychotropics	
Butyrophenones and combinations (Haldol)	causes rash, diarrhea
Hydroxyzines (Vistaril, Atarax)	nursing discouraged; effect unknown
Lithium carbonate	effects unknown, breast-feeding discouraged
Meprobamate and combinations *(Equanil, Miltown)	alternate drug advised
Librium	effects unknown
*Valium	effects unknown; nursing not recommended
Radioisotopes	
I$_{131}$	suppress thyroid gland; all mothers, breast-feeding or not, should not have contact with baby for forty-eight hours
Urinary anti-infectives	
(Bactrim, Septra)	sulfanilamides contraindicated if infant less than two months old
(Thiosulfil, nalidixic acid)	may be noxious if taken continuously
Mandelic acid	photosensitivity, rashes
Vaginals	
AVC creams and other sulfanilamides	
*Flagyl vaginal insert	jaundice of newborn (Gray's syndrome or kernicterus)
*Vaginal douches and gels containing povidone-iodine	possible thyroid problems from high iodine levels

*Especially harmful.

FORMULAS

Infant formulas try to copy the natural composition of human milk. No formula is identical in composition but there are some that come closer than others.

WHAT TO LOOK FOR IN A FORMULA

Soy milk

✤ The Food and Drug Administration has warned parents not to use Eden-soy or similar soy drinks. These are not substitutes for breast milk.

Protein-to-fat ratio

✤ Breast milk has a high-fat, low-protein content to provide enough calories and help in the absorption of iron.

✤ The protein in breast milk is primarily lactalbumin, which is digested by infants.

✤ The protein in formulas is primarily casein, which is not easily digestible.

✤ The brands SMA and PM 60/40 contain the same proteins and protein-to-fat rations as breast milk.

Sugar

✤ Cow's milk formulas add lactose, the natural sugar present in human milk.

✤ Milk-substitute formulas (soy milk) add sucrose.

Mineral content

✤ Only PM 60/40, SMA, and Optimal have a low-soluble amount of minerals similar to breast milk.

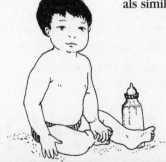

Advantages of bottle feeding

Everyone knows the clear advantages of breast-feeding. Here are some rewards of formula feeding.

→ You're not restricted to the baby by a feeding schedule—you can return to work sooner.

→ You can get more rest; your mate and others can feed the baby.

→ The closeness associated with feeding can be shared by your partner.

→ You can avoid the discomforts of breast-feeding (leaky breasts, sore nipples).

→ Formula may fill the baby up more so she'll go longer between feedings.

→ Not nursing may preserve the shape of your breasts.

WARNINGS!
ABOUT YOUR MILK SUPPLY

✦ The injection given in the hospital to dry up your milk supply is potentially dangerous.

✦ Many hospitals use the hormone DES, which can increase your chances of cancer.

✦ Your milk production will stop by itself if you don't nurse the baby.

✦ You might want to nurse for the first week and then gradually dry up your milk supply.

✦ Studies show that milk supply stops naturally as well as with harmful injections.

SCHEDULE OF SHOTS
FOR THE BABY

* Most pediatricians believe immunizations should be begun at two months of age because they prevent diseases that can take a child's life.
* However, some doctors are now questioning exposure to these powerful medications.
* If you have any questions, discuss them with your doctor. Most doctors follow the immunization schedule below.

IMMUNIZATION CALENDAR

2 months
- ✚ DTP 3-in-1 shot (diphtheria, tetanus, pertussis)
- ✚ Sabin oral live polio vaccine

4 months
- ✚ DTP booster
- ✚ Polio booster

6 months
- ✚ DTP booster

1 year
- ✚ tuberculin test

15 months
- ✚ measles/rubella vaccine
- ✚ mumps vaccine

18 months
- ✚ DTP booster

2 years
- ✚ polio booster
- ✚ Hib vaccine (haemophilus influenza type B)

4 to 6 years
- ✚ DTP booster
- ✚ polio booster

Warning Signs!

Call the Doctor
If Baby Has These Symptoms

- ✤ EXCESSIVE CRYING and unusual irritability
- ✤ EXCESSIVE DROWSINESS; sleeping at times when she or he usually plays
- ✤ POOR SLEEP with frequent waking, restlessness, and crying
- ✤ FEVER with flushed face, hot and dry skin
- ✤ SEVERE LOSS OF APPETITE; refusal to take familiar foods
- ✤ REPEATED VOMITING; throwing up most of a feeding more than once
- ✤ BOWEL MOVEMENTS WITH BLOOD or pus, mucus, a green color, or that are unusually loose or frequent
- ✤ COUGH OR SEVERE RUNNY NOSE
- ✤ INFLAMMATION OR DISCHARGE FROM THE EYES
- ✤ RASH that covers a large portion of the body or persists after changing laundry habits
- ✤ TWITCHING, CONVULSIONS, INABILITY TO MOVE
- ✤ PAIN

14

Your Body
After Childbirth

MISCELLANEOUS BODY
CHANGES

Your breasts

- Your breasts may feel congested.
- You may feel feverish.
- If you are breast-feeding you can hand-express the milk.
- If you are not breast-feeding *do not* hand-express milk, which would stimulate milk production. However, *do* limit your intake of fluids.

Your hair

- Your hair may fall out in greater amounts.
- Hair loss is probably due to a lack of protein, which the placenta was providing.
- Eat plenty of protein-rich foods.
- If your hair is dry or brittle avoid washing it daily.
- Switch to a cream-based shampoo and use a good conditioner.

Getting your period again

- Your period will return anywhere from two to four months after childbirth.
- Most women do not ovulate when they are breast-feeding—but *some do.*
- Don't wait for a period before you resume using birth control. It's possible to ovulate before menstruation.

Your skin

- After childbirth you may have dry skin.
- Breast-feeding women are even more susceptible to dryness; their bodies are using all available fluids for milk production.
- Drink plenty of water.
- Use an oil-based moisturizer.

Your feet

- Your shoe size will probably change to half a size larger after you have a baby.
- This is a *permanent* reminder of pregnancy!
- Don't buy new shoes until after the baby is born unless it's absolutely necessary—they probably won't fit once you're a mother!

Your teeth and gums

- After childbirth you may find your gums inflamed.
- There may be grayness at the gumline of your lower teeth.
- Pregnancy depletes your body of its natural calcium.
- Eat foods rich in calcium and vitamin C.
- Try a soft-bristle toothbrush.

Your uterus

- After childbirth your uterus will feel firm, like a grapefruit in the middle of your stomach.
- It will gradually shrink. By the end of the first week you probably won't be able to feel it when you press on your belly.
- By six weeks after childbirth the uterus should be back to its pre-pregnancy size.

Vaginal discharge (lochia)

- You will have a discharge of blood and mucus for one to six weeks after the birth of your baby.
- If the flow becomes bright red after the first week *notify the doctor.* You will probably be advised to rest.

- Use a sanitary napkin for the first two weeks.
- After two weeks you may use tampons as long as your doctor approves.
- Breast-feeding rapidly reduces the bleeding.
- A continuing vaginal discharge or unpleasant odor may be signs of incomplete healing or infection. Be sure to inform your doctor.

Changes in your vagina

- It will take a couple of weeks for the vagina to resume its usual size and shape.
- Some women's vaginas never return to their pre-pregnant size.
- By doing the Kegel exercise you can tighten your vagina considerably. (The Kegel exercise involves contracting your pelvic muscles, holding the position, and then releasing—repeating the exercise several times. See pages 124–125 for more on Kegels.)
- Your cervix will contract for several weeks after pregnancy.
- You will need to be fitted by your gynecologist for a larger size diaphragm (See "Birth Control" below.)

Your weight

- It is normal to lose ten to twenty pounds immediately after childbirth, depending on how much you gained.
- Although you'll have more weight to lose, do not go on a strict diet for the first month after giving birth.
- Your body needs a nutritious, well-balanced diet to recover from the stress of having a baby.

Birth control

- Don't rely on the fact that you haven't gotten your period.
- You can get pregnant the first time you ovulate: this will be *before* your period occurs.
- Your old diaphragm will not fit *even if you had a cesarean.*
- You'll have to be refitted with a larger size by the doctor about four weeks after giving birth.
- Do not use the pill while breast-feeding.
- Your partner can use condoms with lots of spermicidal foam or jelly.

RECOVERING FROM
THE EPISIOTOMY

The episiotomy is the cut that was made in your perineum (between your anus and vagina) to allow more room for the baby's head.

→ Some women find that recovering from the episiotomy is the most painful part of childbirth.

→ The soreness can last from one to three weeks.

→ Put an ice pack on that area of your vagina soon after giving birth to reduce pain and swelling.

→ Ask your doctor if he recommends anesthetic creams or sprays.

→ Keep your genital area dry and clean.

→ Perineal pads can be put between your sanitary pad and the stitches to relieve itching and soreness.

→ If it's painful to sit, use a soft pillow or a "doughnut cushion."

→ **WARNING:** Do not use any ice or heat treatment if your genitals are already numb from anesthetic spray or cream.

URINATION AND
URINARY TRACT INFECTION

You may have difficulty passing urine after childbirth.

→ Women who do not urinate within six to eight hours after delivery are usually given a catheter.

→ In the first week after delivery you may need to urinate more often because of the extra fluid retained during pregnancy.

→ Urinary tract infections are fairly common after childbirth.

SYMPTOMS OF A
URINARY TRACT INFECTION

Notify your doctor if you think you have an infection so you can take immediate care before it becomes serious. The following symptoms might indicate infection:

✤ Fever

✤ Chills

✤ Discomfort when urinating

✤ Inability to empty the bladder completely

✤ Urinating frequently in small amounts

✤ Abdominal pain or back pain

BOWEL MOVEMENTS AND HEMORRHOIDS

PROBLEMS	ANSWERS
Constipation: You may not be able to have a bowel movement.	■ Drink plenty of liquids and eat a lot of fresh fruit and fiber. ■ Ask your doctor about using a mild laxative; he may recommend an enema, suppositories, or a stool softener. ■ If you are breast-feeding, a stool softener has the same effect as a laxative without affecting your milk.
Hemorrhoids (swollen, tender lumps in your anus) are dilated veins that make bowel movements uncomfortable.	■ Sit in a shallow tub of warm water. ■ Sit on a "doughnut cushion" to avoid discomfort. ■ Your doctor can recommend anesthetic creams or compresses.

WARNING!

CALL DOCTOR IMMEDIATELY IF . . .

- ✤ You have unusually heavy bleeding on any day (more than a menstrual period, or if you soak more than two sanitary napkins in half an hour).
- ✤ You have a vaginal discharge with a strong, unpleasant odor.
- ✤ You have a temperature of 100.4 degrees or higher on any two of the first ten days after birth, not including the first twenty-four hours.
- ✤ After the first day your temperature is 101 or higher.
- ✤ Your breasts are red, feel hot, or are painful.

15.

Bits and Pieces

Rivalry with Siblings (including household pets!)

PREPARING THE BIG BROTHER OR SISTER

The baby-to-be represents a variety of emotional problems for small children you already have.

Why isn't a child delighted about the new baby?

→ It's normal for a child to feel frightened about being abandoned or "traded in" for the new infant.

→ Change can be upsetting.

    ❧ Moving the child's belongings or room.

    ❧ The tumult of creating a new room for the baby.

    ❧ Mommy may not feel well or have her usual energy or patience.

→ Unrealistic expectations that the baby will be an instant playmate are common.

    ❧ This leads to disappointment that all the new baby does is eat and sleep.

    ❧ Disappointment can lead to resentment or hostility.

Making older siblings more comfortable beforehand

→ Make any changes to the child's room as early as possible in your pregnancy to give them time to adjust.

→ Involve your child in setting up the baby's room so he doesn't feel excluded from the planning and changes.

→ Let your child pick out some baby toys and clothes that will be gifts from him to the baby—this allows him to be the generous big brother/sister.

→ So the older sibling will feel special, buy some new things for her room too.

→ Ask what he thinks the baby will look and act like.

    ⮞ This allows him time to prepare mentally for the new arrival.

    ⮞ By discussing a newborn with your child you can allay his fears of being displaced.

→ Some hospitals offer a "Big Brother" and "Big Sister" class for siblings under six years old.

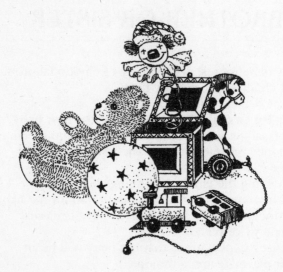

Making your child feel good after the baby arrives

→ Try to maintain his daily rituals.

    ⮞ Try to maintain continuity in his life after the baby arrives.

    ⮞ Regular habits help satisfy a child's need for predictability and routines.

    ⮞ Keep whatever patterns you had set up, like supper/bath/teethbrushing/bedtime story, etc.

→ When the baby cries, ask:
- 🍃 "Do you think the baby feels hungry?"
- 🍃 "Do you think we should change the baby's diaper?"
- 🍃 "Do you think it's hard for the baby that she can't talk to us?"

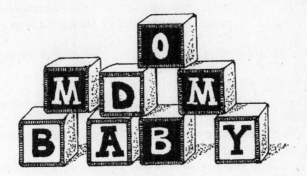

SIBLINGS ATTENDING THE BABY'S BIRTH

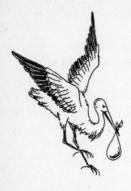

What does this mean for the older child?
→ This practice is often part of a home birth.
→ Having sibling(s) present for the birth is also a choice for couples using an "alternative birthing room" in a hospital or giving birth in a maternity center.

→ Ask the child whether she wants to be there and respect her choice.
- Explain what it will be like.
- Putting pressure on a child can be harmful to her relationship with the baby.

→ Some psychologists believe a child less than five years old is too young to attend the birth.

→ Birth is bloody and messy and you should consider how your child will handle that.

→ You can't predict a child's negative reaction.
- In a child's limited experience your strained expression means anger or pain; blood means injury.
- A bad reaction to birth is more likely if labor is long and difficult.

Suggestions for siblings attending a birth
→ Tell the child as early as possible in your pregnancy that a baby brother or sister is going to be born.

→ Bring the child to at least one prenatal visit.
- Let him listen to the baby's heartbeat.
- By meeting your doctor the child will feel more at ease at the time of delivery.

→ Educate and expose the child to everything possible about the birth process.
- According to his level of understanding, books with diagrams and photos will help explain the process.

→ Show the child a color movie or videotape of a childbirth.
- The experience will be enhanced if he's prepared and knows what to expect.
- Seeing a birth in action can lessen what might otherwise be too intense an experience.

→ Certain topics should be discussed ahead of time with any age child who will be present at the birth:
  ⋅ Blood and amniotic fluid will be on the baby and mother. Reassure the child this is okay, that it happened when she was born too.
  ⋅ Labor is hard work and Mommy can't be interrupted. A child cannot disturb his mother during contractions; he has to let her work.
  ⋅ Mommy's pain is okay. You must explain that the pain is not like when you fall down and get hurt; the pain is good, it's stretching inside and opening to let the baby out.
→ Describe the appearance of the newborn, cord, and placenta.
→ Practice labor and delivery techniques around the child.
→ There should be one adult for each child in attendance.
→ Allow the child to come and go at will from the birth room.
  ⋅ Some children may just not get very interested or involved in the childbirth and there's nothing you can do about it.
→ Don't awaken a sleeping child right at the moment of birth.
  ⋅ If you want to wake him, have a familiar person do it in a calm, reassuring way.
→ Reassure the child immediately after birth, letting him know everything is all right.

Alternatives to having the child present

→ Include the child as much as possible before birth.
  ⋅ Bring the child with you to prenatal exams.
  ⋅ Share any books or other information about pregnancy that a child can understand.
  ⋅ Involve the child in setting up the baby's room and clothes.
→ Introduce the child to the baby as soon as possible.
  ⋅ If you're having an out-of-hospital birth the child can go to a friend's or relative's and return immediately after the baby is born.
  ⋅ Even with a hospital birth you may be able to have your child brought in when the baby is newborn. Check this out ahead of time.
  ⋅ A good time to introduce the sibling may be while you are breast-feeding.
  ⋅ Just bringing the new baby home can create hostility; it would be as though your spouse brought home another woman and announced she was the new "co-wife"!

PETS AND THE NEW BABY

Animals are going to feel jealous

→ Your pets may have been like children for you.
- Many couples "practice parenting" on their pet(s).
- Be compassionate about how displaced your animal(s) must feel to be "thrown over" for a noisy, strange-smelling intruder.
- Take the pet's perspective of the new arrival: you're fussing over a little bundle in the same tone of voice you probably used for the pet(s).

→ You're going to have less time and affection for pet(s) now.
- Your pets may have had a central place in your life before the baby was born.
- It's inevitable that once your baby arrives your pets are going to get less of your emotions.
- This is going to make the animal(s) jealous and set up rivalry with the baby for your affection.

→ Encourage the pet to make friends with the baby.
- Being overprotective will only increase a pet's feeling of jealousy because he's being pushed aside.
- When bringing the baby close to the pet, pat the animal and use an encouraging, gentle tone of voice.
- If the animal sniffs or licks, these are natural reactions: control your knee-jerk reactions to shoo the pet away in protection of the baby.
- Don't reprimand the animal with a harsh tone or strike it.
- Try to see the situation from the animal's point of view: he's confused and displaced.
- Take advantage of the fact that pets generally want to please you.
- Encourage a friendship with the baby with positive reinforcement.

Preparing a pet for the new arrival

→ Get obedience training if your dog doesn't already follow commands.
- You'll need to be able to control and direct your dog when the baby is around.
- You are going to need basic commands like "Sit," "Stay," "Down," "Leave it," "Off," etc.

- You may not feel you have the time or energy to train the dog during pregnancy, but having control may be what allows your dog to make a smooth transition with the baby.

→ Expose your pet(s) to children, especially infants.
  - Encourage people to bring babies to the house: this will familiarize your cat or dog with having an infant on the animal's home turf.
  - Don't worry if your dog is agitated by young children: this doesn't mean there will be a problem with a baby.
  - Youngsters are quite a different adjustment for a pet than an infant. Small children move quickly, talk loudly, and can make motions and sounds that are threatening and startling to pets.

→ Bring a baby doll home and pretend it's real.
  - Put a baby doll in the crib, hold it in your arms, and talk to it as you would a real baby.
  - This will accustom your dog to what's ahead. (Don't let any friends see you doing this or they'll think you're off your rocker!)

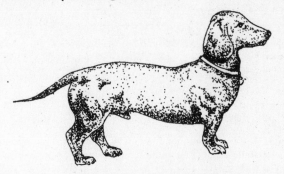

Once the baby comes home

→ Acquaint the dog or cat with your baby's scent.
  - Bring home a receiving blanket or piece of clothing that has been used on your newborn baby.
  - Sense of smell is vital to a dog; this is an important "first introduction."

→ Make an effort to include the pet as much as possible once the baby joins the family.
  - New parents have a tendency to push a pet away.
  - You haven't got as much time for the animal now and you're feeling protective toward the baby.
  - Spurning the pet only increases the animal's feeling of being displaced or rejected.

→ Get new toys or chew bones for a dog.
- Give the dog a treat in the beginning when he's around the baby.
- Consider it a bribe, or a positive reinforcement; the dog will associate the baby with something he likes!

→ Observe the pet around the baby.
- Some dogs become protective and nurturant of the newborn.
- Other pets may feel antagonistic.
- If the dog seems hostile, be wary: look for a tail that is held down and doesn't wag, flattened ears, or more overt hostility like growling or bristling hair.
- To be safe, at least in the early weeks, don't leave any pet alone with the newborn: close the nursery door and/or always have a person around.
- There are some pets, particularly older ones, that may not be able to welcome the baby and make accommodation. But give the animal every opportunity first.

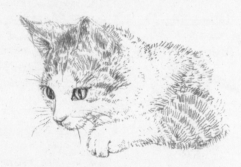

Are pets unhealthy for babies?

→ Household pets do pick up dirt and germs from the ground.
- It's best not to have them in nose-to-nose contact with the infant.

→ Cats often like to make a nest in the crib or bassinet.
- You don't want your baby to sleep on a blanket of cat hairs!
- You can close the cat out of the room with the baby's things in it.
- You can also cover the baby's bed with anti-insect gauzy netting sold for cribs or a similar mesh netting made especially to keep cats out.

Index

A

Abdominal pain, 92, 118
  after cesarean section, 238
Abortion, spontaneous
  see Miscarriage
Accutane, avoiding, 11
Ace inhibitors, avoiding, 11
Acetaminophen, 101
Aerosol ribavirin, avoiding, 11
Aerosol sprays, effects, 25
Age, maternal, and C-section,
  235
Airplane travel, 149–150
Air pollution, 25
Alcohol
  avoiding, 3
  during pregnancy, avoiding,
    10
  effects of, 3
  fetal alcohol syndrome, 10
  sperm, dangers to, 24
Allergies, 92–93
Alpha fetoprotein testing
  (AFP), 121
Alternative birthing centers
  (ABCs), 161, 164
Alveoli, development in fetus,
  77
Amnesics, use during labor, 215
Amniocentesis, 119, 245

Amniotic fluid, 77
  excess (polyhydramnios),
    261
Amniotic sac, rupture of
  see Rupture of membranes
Amphetamines, effects, 10
Analgesics
  and breast-feeding, 283
  labor pain, use to relieve,
    214, 215
Anemia, Cooley's, 30
Anesthetic gases, avoiding, 11,
  25
Anesthetics, use during labor,
  214, 216–218
Anitimetabolites, avoiding,
  12
Ankles, swollen, 112
Antacids, and breast-feeding,
  283
Antibiotics, avoiding, 11, 283
Antibodies, baby in womb, 87
Anticonvulsants, avoiding, 12,
  284
Antihistamines, avoiding, 12
Anxieties, 180–181
  see also Fears about parenting
Apgar rating, newborn, 225
Areola, darkening of, 96, 109
Artificial colors in foods,
  dangers, 51
Aspirin, avoiding, 12, 101
Asthma, 253

B

Baby, 269
  bedding needs, 277
  clothes, 278
  crib, requirements for,
    276-277
  dangers to babies and small
    children, 228-230
  exercise equipment for, 278
  exercise programs for, 227
  feeding, 280
  immunization, 289
  premie, 264-265
  room, baby's, 276
  supplies for, 277
  warning signs, when to call
    doctor, 290
  see also Newborn
Babysitters, 175
Backache, 94
  during labor, 209-210
Barbiturates
  and breast-feeding, 284
  use during labor, 215
Bath support rings, danger to
  babies, 229-230
Bedding needs, baby, 277
Beer, effects, 10
Bicycling, during pregnancy,
  127
Birth control
  after childbirth, 293
  when to stop using, 23
Birth control pills, 12, 23
Birth defects, 30-32
  birth control methods and,
    23
  caffeine and, 3

everyday hazards, 25-29
genetic defects, 30
listeriosis as cause, 37
medications and, 3, 11-14
prenatal diagnosis, see Prenatal diagnosis
"street drugs," effects of, 10
vitamin supplements and,
  22
Birthing chair, 222
Bladder
  infection, 114
  in pregnancy, 113
Bleeding, 95, 118
  heavy, postpartum, 296
  nosebleeds, 106
  rectal bleeding, 103
  and spotting, 95, 118
  after sexual intercourse, in
    first three months,
    136-137
Blood-pressure-lowering
  drugs, 11, 13
Blood tests
  preconception, 2
  purpose of, 122
  for rubella, 31
  when done, 122
Bloody show, prelabor sign,
  204, 207
Body changes, during pregnancy, 95
  sex and, 129
Body changes, postpartum,
  291-293
Bonding to baby, 226
Bottle-feeding, 288
Bowel movements
  after cesarean section, 238
  and hemorrhoids, 295
  newborn, 272

Bradley method of childbirth,
165
Brain, development of fetus's,
64–65, 71, 86
Braxton-Hicks contractions,
204
Breast-feeding, 281–282
advantages, 281
after cesarean section, 238
hospital policy, finding out,
157–158
lactation consultants, 282
medications to avoid,
283–286
nutrition, 281
preparation for, 281
sexual stimulation,
increased, 139
sore nipples, 282–283
Breast milk
jaundice, 275
leakage, 140
production of milk, 288
Breasts
cancer, screening during
pregnancy, 96
changes, postpartum, 291,
296
pregnancy bras, 96
swelling, 95–96
Breathing, baby in womb, 86,
88
Breathlessness, 108
Breech birth, 257
Breech presentation
causes for, 258
cesarean section, 234
dangers, 259
positions, different types of,
258
vaginal delivery, 259

Brewer's yeast, 16
Brown spots, skin problems,
109

C

Cadmium, effects, 25
Caffeine, 25
before pregnancy, avoiding,
3
in chocolate, 9
in coffee, 9
cutting down on, 8
during pregnancy, 8
and fetal death, 8
in nonprescription drugs,
9
in soft drinks, 9
in tea, 9
Calcium
dietary sources, 19, 43–44
importance of, 41
supplements, 19
vegetarians, possible deficiencies for, 60
Vitamin C and, 42
Vitamin D and, 42
Calisthenics, during pregnancy,
127
Cancer chemotherapy, effects,
12
drugs for chemotherapy, 16
Carbon monoxide, avoiding,
25
Cardiovascular preparations,
and breast-feeding, 284
Carpal tunnel syndrome, 107

Cooley's anemia, 30
Cortisone, effects, 12
Cough preparations, and
    breast-feeding, 284
Cough syrup, effects, 12
Crack, effects, 10
Cramps
    muscle cramps, 104
Crib, requirements for,
    276–277
Crib toys, danger to babies,
    230
Crying
    baby in womb, 81
    newborn, 273, 290
C-section
    see Cesarean section
Cystic fibrosis, 30
Cystitis (bladder infection),
    114

D

Dairy products
    as calcium source, 43–44
    as protein source, 46
    intolerance, 42, 97–98
    see also Milk
Danger signs during preg-
    nancy, 118
Defects, birth
    see Birth defects
Dehydration caused by vomit-
    ing, 117
Delivery
    see Labor
Demerol, 214

Dental checkups, preconcep-
    tion, 2
Depression, postpartum,
    182–185
Diabetes, in pregnancy,
    249–250
Diet
    breast-feeding mothers,
        281–282
    herpes simplex virus, role in
        controlling, 36
    pre-pregnancy, 3
    vegetarian, 55–60
    vitamins, dietary sources
        and supplements, 3,
        15–22
Dieting before pregnancy, 2
Diet pills, effects, 13
Dilation, 207–208, 210
Discharge from hospital, 158
Diseases, infectious, harm to
    baby, 35–38
Diuretics
    and breast-feeding, 285
    effects, 13, 112
Dizziness, 98, 108, 118
Doctor
    complete checkup before
        pregnancy, 2
    false labor, calling doctor,
        205
    questions to ask, 154–156
    selecting, 154–156
    travel, consulting doctor,
        148
    when to call, 206
Domestic help, 175
Dorsal position, for labor,
    221
Douching, and vaginal dis-
    charge, 115

Dreams, in pregnancy,
186–187
Drugs, 3, 10
see also Medications

E

Ectopic pregnancy, 118, 249
Edema (swelling), 111–112
Electromagnetic fields exposure, danger to sperm, 24
Emergency delivery, 242–244
Emotions
and cesarean section, 237
and childbirth, 169–201,
219
Enemas in labor, 159
Engagement, prelabor sign,
201
Epidural anesthesia, 214, 217
Episiotomy, 224
local infiltration of, 218
recovering from, 294
Excess energy, 204
Exercise equipment for baby,
278
Exercise programs for babies,
227
Exercises, before pregnancy, 2
Exercises, during pregnancy,
124–128
best exercises, 127
breech presentation, 259
Kegel exercises, 103,
124–125
safe exercise, guidelines,
124–125

swelling, to relieve, 112
warnings, 126, 128
worst exercises, 127
External genitals, newborn,
271–272
Eyes
development of fetus's, 66,
69, 82, 85
newborn, 271

F

Face masks, use of during
delivery, 212
Facial expressions, baby in
womb, 72
Faintness, 98, 108
False labor, 205
Family attending birth, 164,
300–301
Family-centered maternity
care, 157, 164
Father
adjustment to parenthood,
195–196
disinterest, 199
envy and jealousy, 198
fears, 196
jealousy, 198
motherly feelings, 198
new-age dads, 195
nurturant feelings, 198
practice for parenting,
198
preparation for parental
role, 199
becoming workaholic, 201

Grains, as protein source, 47,
56
Groin pains, 100
Gums
care of, 113
changes, postpartum, 292

H

Hair
baby in womb, 74–75, 87,
89
changes, during pregnancy,
100–101
changes, postpartum, 291
lanugo, 89
Haldol, effects, 13
Hands, swollen, 112
Hands-and-knees position, for
labor, 222
Hard liquor, effects, 10
Headaches, 101–102, 118
Head-down position, baby in
womb
see Vertex position, baby in
womb
Hearing, baby in womb, 74, 76,
80, 83
Heart, development of fetus's,
66–69, 73
Heartburn, 102
Hemorrhoids, 103, 295
Hepatitis B, 35
Heroin, effects, 10
Herpes simplex virus, 35–36,
257

Hiccups, baby in womb,
81, 93
High blood pressure, 251–252
High-salt foods, and swelling,
112
Hormones, 285
Horseback riding, during preg-
nancy, 127
Hospital
choosing, 157–159
coping with, 160
what to take to, 205
Hot tubs, effects, 26
Household cleaning products,
effects, 26
Hunger, after birth, 213
Hyperemesis gravidarum, 117,
118
Hypertension, 251–252

I

Ibuprofen, 101
Identical twins, 260
Immunization
baby, 289
during pregnancy, 31
Indigestion, 102
Infants
see Baby; Newborn
Infectious diseases, harm to
baby, 35–38
Inhalation analgesia, use dur-
ing labor, 215
Intercourse, sexual
see Sexual intercourse

Intravenous drip, during labor, 159
Iodides, effects, 13
Iodine
   dietary sources and supplements, 20
   vegetarians, possible deficiencies for, 60
Iron, 48–49
   absorption of, increasing, 48
   deficiency, 48
   dietary sources, 15, 20–21, 49
   supplements, 15, 20–21, 48
   vegetarians, possible deficiencies for, 60
Isolation, after pregnancy, 164
Itchy stomach, 103–104

J

Jaundice, baby, 275
Jogging, during pregnancy, 127
Juices, as iron source, 49

K

Kegel exercises, 103, 124–125
Kicking, baby, 93–94
   see also Fetal movement
Kidney infection, 114

L

Labor
   active phase, 207–208
   backache during, 209–210
   cesarean section, indications before labor, 234
   coaching, early labor, 219–220
   delivery table, transfer to, 212
   examination during, 210
   father's participation in, 199
   first-stage, 207–210, 219–220
   inducing, 214, 216
   medications used during, 214–215
   pain medications, 214
   placenta, delivery of, 213
   positions, 221–222
   premature, 118, 264–265
   psychological aspects, 219
   pushing stage, 211
   second-stage, 211–212
   speeding up, 214, 216
   stages of, 207–213
   third-stage, 213
   transition phase, 208–209, 223
   urge to push, 211, 242
   when to call doctor, 206
   see also Childbirth
Lactation consultants, 282
Lactose intolerance, 42
Lamaze, 160, 165
Lanugo hair, baby in womb, 89

Moving, during pregnancy,
    considerations, 145–147
Mucus, increased vaginal, 204
Muscle cramps, 104
Muscle relaxants, and breast-
    feeding, 285

N

Nails, care of, 100
Narcotics, use during labor,
    215
Nausea, 105–106, 118
Neural tube defects, 31
Newborn, 225–226
    appearance, 270–272
    bonding to baby, 226
    bowel movements, 272
    cesarean baby, 237
    circulation and tempera-
      ture, 272
    circumcision, 144, 274
    crying, 273
    emergency delivery, 244
    external genitals, 271–272
    eyes, 272
    head, 272
    jaundice, 275
    reflexes, 272
    skin, 270
    temperature, 272
    umbilical cord stump, 272
    see also Baby
Niacin, dietary sources and
    supplements, 17
Nightmares, in pregnancy,
    188

Nose
    nosebleeds, 106
    stuffy nose, 110–111
Nose drops and sprays, effects,
    13
Nuts and seeds
    as iron source, 49–50
    as protein source, 47, 49

O

Obesity and pregnancy, 2
Obstetrician
    see Doctor
Orgasms, 134–135
Overheating, in pregnancy,
    106–107
Over-the-counter medications,
    avoiding, 3
Oxytocin challenge test, 245
Oxytocins, use to induce or
    speed labor, 214, 216
Ozone, effects, 27

P

Paints
    dangers, 27
    regular exposure to, danger
      to sperm, 24
Pap smears, preconception, 2
Paracervical block (anesthesia),
    218

PCBs, avoiding, 27
Pediatrician, selecting, 144
Pesticides, dangers, 28
Pets, and new baby, 302–304
Phenacetin, effects, 13
Photographic chemicals, dangers, 28
Photographs, at hospital, 158
Physical examinations, preconception, 2
Pins and needles in hands and feet, experiencing, 107
Piper forceps, 259
Placenta
    abruptio, 118, 233, 262
    delivery of, 213, 244
    examination of, 213
    function of, 73
    pervia, 233, 262
    third-stage labor, 213
Polyhydramnios (excess amniotic fluid), 261
Positions
    for intercourse during pregnancy, 136
    for labor, 136
Postpartum body changes, 291–294
    warnings, when to call doctor, 296
Postpartum depression, 182–185
Post-term delivery, 234
Preconception checkups, 2
Prelabor signs, 201
Premature labor, 118, 264–265
Prenatal diagnosis
    alpha fetoprotein testing (AFP), 121
    amniocentesis, 119
    blood tests, see Blood tests

cell tests, 122
chorionic villus sampling (CVS), 120
ultrasound, 121
Prenatal education classes, at hospital, 158
Preparation, preconception, 2
Preregistration at hospital, 158
Prescription medications, avoiding, 3
Progestins, effects, 13
Prolapsed cord, 233, 242
Protein
    dietary sources, 45–47
    in vegetarian diet, 55–58
Psychotropics, and breast-feeding, 285
Pudendal block (anesthesia), 218
Pushing stage of childbirth, 211
Pyelitis (kidney infection), 114

R

Radioisotopes, avoiding, 285
Recovery room, 213
Recreational drugs, avoiding, 3
Rectal bleeding, 103
Red meat, hormones and antibiotics in, dangers, 51
Reflexes, newborn, 272
Relocation, during pregnancy, considerations, 145–147
REM (rapid eye movement), fetus's, 81
Reserpine, effects, 13

Vitamin C
  calcium and, 42
  dietary sources, 16, 18–19, 22
  sperm, deficiency causing
    damage to, 24
  supplements, 16, 18–19
Vitamin D
  calcium and, 42
  dietary sources, 19, 22
  supplements, 19, 22
  vegetarians, possible defi-
    ciencies for, 60
Vitamin E, dietary sources and
    supplements, 20, 22
Vitamin K, dietary sources and
    supplements, 21, 22
Vitamins
  caution in using supple-
    ments, 14, 22
  daily requirement, 16
  dietary sources, 16–21
  purpose of, 16
  same daily amount of sup-
    plements, 22
  see also individual vitamins
Vomiting, 117, 118
  see also Nausea

W

Walking, during pregnancy, 127
Water, 28
  drinking in pregnancy, 2
  filters on tap, using, 6
  lead in, protecting yourself
    from, 4–6, 27
  testing, 4–5
  well water, 4–5

Waterbeds, danger to babies
    and small children, 229
Week-by-week development,
    63–89
Weight, baby's
  marijuana effects on, 10
  smoking effects on, 7
Weight gain, 40
  breakdown of, 40
  sudden, 118
  toxemia, 118
  Varicose veins, excessive
    weight gain and, 116
Weight loss, 204, 293
Wilson's disease, 34
Wine, effects, 10
Worries, 180–181

X

X-rays, avoiding, 2, 29

Y

Yeast infection, during preg-
    nancy, 254
Yogurt as calcium source, 44

Z

Zinc, dietary sources and sup-
    plements, 21